Springer Series on the Teaching of Nursing

Diane O. McGivern, RN, PhD, FAAN, Series Editor
New York University Division of Nursing

Advisory Board: *Ellen Baer, PhD, RN, FAAN; Carla Mariano, EdD, RN; Janet A. Rodgers, PhD, RN, FAAN; Alice Adam Young, PhD, RN*

Barbara Carty, RN, EdD, FAAN, received her doctorate from the Teachers College, Columbia University. Her main area of research addressed "The Information Needs of Nurses in The Acute Care Setting." She is actively involved in informatics research, including the development of an Electronic Data Repository within the Mt. Sinai, New York Health consortium and the Nursing Care Quality Data Committee of the NYU/Mt. Sinai Health and LIJ/North Shore Alliance. Dr. Carty currently serves on the New York Medical Society Informatics Task Force on Quality Care, and the Advisory Board of "Bridging the Digital Divide" sponsored by National Cancer Institute and Cancer Information Service.

Dr. Carty has served on a number of review panels, including the American Medical Informatics Association and the National Library of Medicine. She has been the recipient of privately funded grants for informatics and education, including interactive web development for home monitoring of patients.

She developed the graduate program in nursing informatics at NYU and is currently Clinical Associate Professor and Coordinator of the Informatics Program at New York University.

NURSING INFORMATICS
EDUCATION FOR PRACTICE

Barbara Carty, RN, EdD, FAAN

 *Springer Series on the
Teaching of Nursing*

Springer Publishing Company, Inc.
536 Broadway
New York, NY 10012-3955

Acquisitions Editor: Ruth Chasek
Production Editor: Janice Stangel
Cover design by Susan Hauley

Library of Congress Cataloging-in-Publication Data

Nursing informatics : education for practice / Barbara Carty, editor
    p. ;   cm. (Springer series on the teaching of nursing)
  Includes bibliographical references and index.
  ISBN 0-8261-1356-7 (hardcover)
    1. Nursing informatics.   2. Nursing—Study and teaching.   I. Carty, Barbara.
  II. Springer series on the teaching of nursing (Unnumbered)
    [DNLM: 1. Education, Nursing.   2. Medical Informatics—education.   WY 18
    N9739 2000]
  RT50.5 .N8695 2000
  610.73'071—dc21   00-030137

Printed in the United States of America

To all nursing informatics students
who are truly pioneers and will bring major changes to
health care and the nursing profession.

Contents

Contributors

Suzanne Bakken, R.N., DNSc, FAAN
Professor
School of Nursing and Medical Informatics
Columbia University
New York, New York

Ginger C. Bjornstad, M.S., R.N.
Senior Clinical Analyst
Intermountain Health Care
Salt Lake City, Utah

Carole A. Gassert, Ph.D., R.N.
Informatics Nurse Consultant
Division of Nursing
Bureau of Health Professions
Distance Learning Advisor
Office for the Advancement of Telehealth
Health Resources and Services Administration
Rockville, Maryland

Linda Goodwin, Ph.D., R.N.
Duke University
Director, Nursing Informatics Program
Division Chief, School of Nursing Health Systems Leadership & Outcomes
Joint Appointments: Information Services and Community & Family Medicine
Durham, North Carolina

Judith Graves Ph.D., R.N.
Scholar-in-Residence
Sigma Theta Tau, International
Indianapolis, Indiana

John P. Lussier, B.S.N., R.N.
Application Specialist
Intermoutain Health Care
Palm Springs, California

Catherine O. Mallard, M.Ed., R.N.
Director, Clinical Systems Design
Visiting Nurse Service of New York
New York, New York

Susan Matney, M.S., R.N.
Medical Vocabulary Engineer
Intermountain Health Care
Salt Lake City, Utah

Susanne Miller, M.S., R.N.
Nursing Informatics Specialist
Intermoutain Health Care
Salt Lake City, Utah

Nancy C. Nelson, B.S.N., R.N.
Clinical Information Systems Coordinator
LDS Hospital
Salt Lake City, Utah

Mig Neiswanger, A.D., B.S.N., R.N.
Clinical Information Systems
  Coordinator
McKay-Dee Hospital Center
Ogden, Utah

Karen Pinto, B.S.N., R.N.
IHC Clinical Operations
  Leader/IS Coordinator for
  the Oncology Clinical
  Program
Intermountain Health Care
Salt Lake City, Utah

Diane Skiba, Ph.D.
Associate Professor
School of Nursing
University Colorado
Denver, Colorado

Nancy Staggers, Ph.D., R.N.
Associate Professor, Clinical
  Informatics
College of Nursing
University of Utah
Salt Lake City, Utah

Cheryl Bagley Thompson, PhD., R.N.
Associate Professor
University of Nebraska College
  of Nursing
Omaha, Nebraska

James P. Turley, Ph.D., R.N.
Vice-chair and Associate
  Professor
Department of Health
  Informatics
University of Texas-Houston
Houston, Texas

Diana Willson, M.S., R.N.
Clinical Analyst/Screen
  Designer
Intermountain Health Care
Salt Lake City, Utah

Rita D. Zielstorff, R.N., M.S., FAAN, FACMI
HEALTHvision
Waltham, Massachusetts

Preface

The need for nursing to keep apace of the rapid changes in society is paramount if we are to continue to make a difference in health care and maintain the relevancy of our profession. The rapid advances taking place in the development and application of information technology in today's society are unparalleled. As a result, we communicate, relate, work, and take our leisure in ways that are intensely interconnected and interactive.

Teaching, the purview of educators, is no less affected by the tumultuous changes taking place in society. Therefore, it is timely for a book on nursing informatics that encompasses both education and practice. It is hoped that the discussions and presentations in this book will become common practice in the teaching arena and practice setting within the next few years. For we have no time to spare in the adoption of new technologies, concepts and strategies into our profession.

Educators as well as students of nursing informatics will discover many new and relevant ideas and strategies to incorporate into their teaching and practice milieu. Computer literacy, information management, nursing taxonomies and standards, web-based teaching strategies, and the electronic patient record are a sampling of the topics addressed in the text. The emerging role of nurses as system analysts, designers, developers and implementers are described in detail as are various education and research models. The final chapter, "Informatics and Education: The Start of a Discussion," brings the presentations full circle and poses questions and challenges to educators, students and practitioners.

The contributors to this text are experts in the field of nursing informatics and represent a variety of perspectives in education, research and practice. They present innovative and creative approaches to conceptualizing, teaching, and implementing the evolving domain of nursing informatics. They are the innovators in a field that has the potential for shaping and altering the nursing profession in profound ways. I am deeply indebted to them for sharing their knowledge, research and practice expertise with the current generation of nurses who are grappling with the myriad of innovations and changes within their profession and society in general.

Barbara Carty

1

Nursing Informatics:
Preparing Nurses for an Evolving Role
Barbara Carty

What little time is left in this century is rehearsal for the chief psychological chore of the 21st century: letting go.—Kelly (1994)

Preparing nurses for the challenges in the rapidly evolving world of health care delivery is a daunting task. In this millennium, health care is dominated by the emergence of enterprise systems, electronic communications, including the computerized patient record (CPR), health care portals, and the replacement, in some cases, of brick and mortar hospitals with virtual delivery systems. The health care industry will be permanently affected as on-line consumer health care markets expand and E-commerce networks develop. Internet technologies will dominate the industry. By 2003, it is anticipated that Internet consumer health care transactions will grow to $1.7 billion (McGeady, 1999). In addition, the information technology (IT) health care market is expected to grow from $13.6 billion in 1997 to $21 billion by 2000 (Essex, 1999). A recent poll conducted by Harris found that 68% of on-line adults seek health information indicating that health care will be strongly influenced by Internet health portals and interactive health information networks.

The impetus for this accelerated access to and availability of information has been the development and introduction of the World Wide Web (WWW) into homes, offices, businesses, and health care settings. Internet-based health care networks linking caregivers and patients provide customized health tools and E-commerce to patients, thus enabling patients to monitor their health status, report health data, access disease prevention information, purchase health care products, and influence health outcomes.

What does this tell us about the role of nurses in the 21st century? The rapid changes taking place will alter the role of health care providers as patients access their records on-line and become managers of their own health. In the electronic environment, societal changes and the effects of consumer informatics on health care will shape the nurse-patient relationship. Patients and providers will work in a more collaborative manner and health care decisions will be made jointly. But more importantly, many issues are on the horizon that will require innovative thinking and problem solving by nurses.

In addition, nurses and other health care providers will have to possess knowledge and experience in health informatics with a specific emphasis on nursing informatics in the nursing curricula. Ideally, basic informatics content should be embedded in all nursing curricula, with advanced specialization on the graduate levels. On a generic level nursing informatics encompasses information science, computer science, and nursing science.

There are driving forces propelling both the changes in education and the role of health care providers in an information-intensive society. The three most prominent factors are 1) the rapid changes of computer-based technology, 2) the continuous evolution of health care financing, and 3) the emerging and changing roles of health care professionals and consumers.

Following a discussion of the technology environment in health care, the area of informatics will be presented as it relates to the education and preparation of the health care practitioner, specifically the nurse, and finally, the position of nursing and the role of nurses in an information-intensive era will be reviewed.

THE HEALTH INFORMATION ENVIRONMENT FOR 2000

It is not possible to talk about the rapidly changing innovations in health care technology without including the major shifts occurring in the health care system, which are both propelled and enhanced by technology. The development of sophisticated information technology (IT) networks, the expansion of integrated delivery systems (IDS's), and the growth of the electronic patient record (EPR) are the outcomes of both major restructuring and rapid technological development. As a result, health care providers find themselves practicing in an environment that has changed significantly and will continue to do so. Table 1.1 illustrates the paradigm shift in health care resulting from changes in information technology and health care financing.

With the move from stand-alone hospital information systems to integrated delivery networks, the availability of the types, quality, and amount of information will determine how care is delivered, evaluated, and financed. As the system moves to enterprise-based organizations, the role of patients (consumers), providers, and settings will interact to produce a more dynamic, interactive environment which will be dominated by information and data access.

The rapid proliferation of managed care has also spawned an increased demand for information on cost and outcomes. This demand in turn has altered how care is delivered and practiced. Decisions on treatments, information on illness prevention, protocols, and clinical pathways are possible because of the availability of aggregate patient data and data repositories.

As the demand for health information accelerates and the ability to process, store, and retrieve data improves, additional changes in the health care environment can be anticipated. A recent report by the committee on privacy and security in health care underscored three major factors affecting the health care industry: 1) consolidation of providers and mergers of care-financing and provider organizations, 2) sophisticated management systems to analyze and share expenditures, and 3) new players involved in clinical practice and decision making (NAP, 1997). As a result, the electronic medical

TABLE 1.1 Health Care Delivery Paradigm Shift

Traditional System	Information-Driven System
Hospital Information Systems (HIS)	Integrated Delivery Systems (IDS)
Hospital-based	Enterprise-based
Illness focused	Wellness & illness focused
Encounter determined	Comprehensive across continuum
Episodic record	Longitudinal record
Local Area Network (LAN)	World Wide Web (WWW)
Professional focus	Consumer focus

record (EMR) will continue to emerge as a major component in the documenting, tracking, assessing, financing, and researching of care delivery.

Health Information Systems

Hospital information systems have moved from stand-alone, hospital-based local area networks systems to dynamic, interactive, health information enterprise systems supported by integrated delivery systems (IDS). The enterprise system is usually comprised of multiple hospitals, primary care providers, ambulatory centers, long-term care facilities, and home health agencies. Technologically, the IDS supports the operations, communications, and outcomes of the enterprise systems. An IDS is composed of "health care providers, service providers, and facilities organized to provide a continuum of health care services to a defined population" (Dick, Steen, & Detmer, 1997). As a result, users who access these systems have expanded from clinicians to financial managers, insurers, regulatory agencies, patients, and in some cases, pharmaceutical companies and health product organizations.

Computer-Based Patient Record

The original computer patient record, intended to replace the paper record has evolved into "electronically stored information about an individual's lifetime health status and health care." (CPRI, 1995). A more expansive definition states that the computer record is a personal health library providing access to all resources on a patient's health history and insurance information; a linking system rather than an independent database, more a process than a product (Tabar, 1999).

Within the past five years the computerized patient record (CPR) has transformed from a straightforward documentation system to a complex, dynamic electronic medical record (EMR) within enterprise systems. Tang and Hammond (1997) have identified five major hallmarks of the CPR: 1) integrated view of patient data, 2) access to knowledge resources, 3) physician order entry and clinician data entry, 4) integrated communication support, and 5) clinical decision support.

With the increased portability of health care information has come the added responsibility to monitor access, provide security, and institute uniform standards and legislation for electronic health care data. In an attempt to address these issues, the Health Insurance Portability and Accountability Act (HIPAA, 1996) was introduced. Congress failed in the 1999 session to pass specific legislation related to privacy and confidentiality as specified in HIPAA. As a result, the responsibility for regulations will be with the Department of Health and Human Services (DHHS). Currently, the only legislation for the security of patient medical information is provided by individual states. In addition, the National Committee on Vital and Health Statistics (NCVHS) is charged with determining national standards for data exchange in health care records.

With a multitude of requirements inherent in the computerization of health care, the need to develop practitioners knowledgeable in the applications, development, and support of these systems is essential. For the immediate future, all nurses should be required to be informed users of the systems, responsible for understanding the importance of standard language, nursing classification systems, and the basic operation of the systems in everyday practice. In addition, a level of advanced specialists are needed who will design, analyze, implement, and evaluate the systems. These specialists will also be responsible for incorporating standards and outcomes associated with their practice.

INFORMATICS, HEALTH CARE, AND EDUCATION

The area of informatics in health care has been undergoing rapid changes in the past decade. Although informatics is a new specialty, the demand for qualified professionals will continue to increase. It is projected that computer and data processing and health services will experience the fastest employment growth over the next 10 years. The projected employment growth will be 108% in the computer industry and 68% in health services (Department of Labor, 1999). This increase underscores the need for qualified health care professionals to 1) be proficient in the management of health care data, and 2) be able to work with computer specialists to design effective health care systems. In our "point and click" society, professionals who do not have a basic understanding of integrated networks and automated patient care records will be at a distinct disadvantage in their ability to maintain the relevancy of their practice. The accelerated development and use of technology in health care delivery has prompted the demand for health care professionals, specifically physicians and nurses, to develop expertise in the application of automated delivery systems. It has also spawned the need for professionals to examine their domains and develop standard vocabulary, patient care protocols, and outcomes for incorporation into electronic systems for storage, documentation, retrieval, and research. As a result, nurses, physicians, and other health care providers have had to articulate their domain of informatics.

Shortliffe and Greenes (1990) defined medical informatics as the "scientific field that deals with the storage, retrieval, and optimal use of biomedical information, data, and knowledge for problem solving and decision making." In 1989, Corcoran and Graves, defined nursing informatics as the "Management and processing of nursing data into nursing information, and nursing data and information into nursing knowledge for the purpose of patient care." In 1994, the American Nursing Association (ANA) further defined the scope of nursing informatics practice as the specialty that "integrates nursing science, computer science, and information science in identifying, collecting, processing, and managing data and information to support nursing practice, administration, education, research and the expansion of nursing knowledge." The position of ANA was a direct outcome of efforts by proponents of nursing informatics to have it recognized as a specialty within nursing. The acknowledgement of nursing informatics is crucial to the advancement and relevancy of the profession within an ever-expanding digital dominated health care system.

The preparation of practitioners, faculty, and students, however, in the area of informatics remains a challenge to the profession. The explication and articulation of nursing's language and vocabulary in both education and practice is a relatively new field and one that has been greatly informed and advanced with the development of informatics. Nursing language is the set of characters, conventions, and rules used to convey ideas and information (Lang et al, 1995). There have been major efforts by researchers to champion the recognition of nursing informatics by developing nursing taxonomies, language and classification systems, and designing clinical systems that reflect patient outcomes and effective nursing interventions (Bakken,

Cashen, & O'Brien, 1999; Clark, 1997; Grobe, 1996; Henry & Mead, 1997; Maas, Johnson, & Mooched, 1996; McCormick, 1994; NCNR, 1993; Zielstorff, 1995). Much remains to be accomplished, however, in the work of decision support, consumer informatics, and the incorporation of nursing terminology into computer-based systems. Paralleling the refinement of nursing language to reflect interventions and outcomes is the need to educate the vast majority of nurses, faculty, and students in basic nursing informatics content as well as specialists with a comprehensive and advanced perspective of the specialty. The formidable task is to continue to develop the specialized area of nursing informatics, while contributing to the interdisciplinary efforts within the broader area of health informatics.

An Interdisciplinary Model

The emergence of informatics as a multidisciplinary entity is a natural outgrowth of the current emphasis on interdisciplinary health care delivery models and integrated networks. In support of this concept, the 1999 American Medical Informatics Association Spring Congress on "Health Informatics Education" sponsored two days of sessions on the future of health informatics education, with special emphasis on interdisciplinary courses and curricula. The presenters represented a number of disciplines including: medicine, nursing, engineering, information management, patient education, and cognitive and library science. The outcome of the sessions supported a professional education model with an interdisciplinary focus. This marked the beginning of a dialogue on an interdisciplinary model of education in health informatics. What does this portend for nursing and specifically nursing informatics?

It is clearly supported that nursing informatics has a specific nursing focus, but there are acknowledged areas of interdisciplinary and collaborative foci that need to be explored and studied (Patel & Kaufman, 1998; Ribbons, 1998; Turley, 1996).

In addition, since the model of Corcoran and Graves was originally postulated tremendous advances and changes have taken place in both health care delivery and technology development. These changes have had a direct effect on promoting the discipline of health informatics. As a result, the emphasis on an interdisciplinary model of health care informatics has assumed even more prominence.

(Gassert, 1998; Greenes & Lorenzi, 1998; Stead, 1998, 99). Nursing, then, has to continue to identify the domain of nursing informatics, still in its infancy, while contributing to and collaborating with the emerging discipline of health informatics.

AN EVOLVING ROLE

The emergence of a health care system dominated by data-driven decisions, managed care, and information technology is affecting the roles of health care providers in both obvious and subtle ways. Managed care's emphasis on an interdisciplinary model of delivery is driving the collaboration of professionals as well as patients to define effective processes and improve clinical outcomes. Physicians refer to "patient-centered" care, nurses prescribe treatments and medications in primary care settings, and patients choose treatment regimes based on consumer ratings. Boundaries, which in the past were clearly defined, are now merging and providing a landscape where professionals and patients are navigating for the first time. This trend will continue as the need to manage and deliver information becomes an essential component of education and health care. As a result, all nurses will need to incorporate new and innovative strategies into their everyday practice. The inclusion of computer-mediated interventions, technology-based communications, and data-driven decisions will become part of everyday practice for all nurses, not only the informatics specialist.

The discipline of informatics clearly illustrates the rapidly shifting landscape. Nurse informatics specialists are charting new territory as they work with peers to design, analyze, and evaluate clinical systems. They collaborate with other health care professionals as well as programmers, information management teams and system designers (Gassert, 1998; HRSA, 1997). They are in many instances learning "on the job," and creating new positions and job descriptions in an information intensive industry (Arnold, 1996; Carty, 1994).

As computer hardware and software becomes even more ubiquitous, the ability to manage data and information and represent knowledge will continue to influence how clinicians practice and how health outcomes are measured.

The incorporation of decision support systems into clinical systems and the ability to access knowledge sources and research repositories will provide users with sophisticated knowledge systems that have the potential to dramatically alter the delivery and outcomes of care. The communication and collaborative capability of information technology will have the effect of producing seamless, interactive systems that will support knowledge representation, facilitate human interaction, and provide new avenues for research in both practice and education.

The role of the nurse informaticist will continue to expand, the specialty will demand credentialing on a graduate level, and the specialist will assume a prominent role in the new paradigm of health care delivery and research.

Role Diversity

The increasing numbers of practicing nurses who are employed outside the traditional hospital setting supports further evidence of the shift in health care delivery.

The latest registered nurse survey indicates that 40% of nurses work outside of a hospital setting with a majority employed in community and ambulatory settings (HRSA, 1996). In addition, more nurses are seeking credentials for independent practice roles and schools are graduating increasing numbers of advanced nurse practitioners. The latest data from the American Nurses Credentialing Center (ANCC) indicates an all-time high of credentialed nurse practitioners for 1998–99: pediatrics, 3,053; adult, 1,427; family nurse, 21,124; gerontology, 3,206; and acute care, 1,574. (ANCC, 1999). It is in these independent practice environments that nurses will rely on information access, data transfer, and innovative patient interaction and communication systems for accountable and measurable care and outcomes.

As nurses and other health professionals find themselves in nontraditional settings, the challenge will be to develop systems which will capture health care encounters and the outcomes of the encounters. Nurses will have to work with their colleagues in informatics, information systems, and computer technology to create systems, which are capable of storing, collecting and analyzing the data.

Essential to the collection and analysis of patient data is the development and adoption of standard terms to structure the data so care may be documented and its effectiveness evaluated. To this end, a number of nurse informatics researchers have developed standard terminology which have been recognized by the American Nurses Association (1998) as acceptable for inclusion in the patient care record. These vocabularies include the : 1) Patient Care Data Set (PCDS), 2) Home Health Care Classification (HHCC), 3) Omaha system, 4) North American Nursing Diagnosis Association (NANDA), 5) Nursing Intervention Classification (NIC), 5) Nursing Outcomes Classification (NOC), 6) the Perioperative Nursing Dataset, 8) Nursing Management Minimum Data Set (NMMDS), and 7) SNOMED RT. (*http://nursingworld.org/nidsec/index.htm*)

The classification systems are an important step in assuring that the language of nursing will be included in the health data records and that health outcomes will be correlated with nursing activities. However, it is equally important that these vocabularies are included in nursing curricula and faculty, students, and practicing nurses understand their importance in defining the care they administer and evaluate.

In addition to the need to create and endorse standard vocabularies in nursing, current and past literature reveal enormous efforts by nurse informaticists to develop, design, and research nursing specific as well as interdisciplinary areas of decision support for patient care data. Specialists in nursing informatics have expanded their work with interdisciplinary teams to develop sophisticated programs for decision support, interactive multimedia health care and telehealth delivery systems (Brennan, Moore, & Caldwell, 1999; Lindberg, 1997; Zielstorff, 1997; 1998). This new area in nursing will grow as our society relies on essential information systems to deliver, research, and teach health care.

As a consequence of the shifts in the health care delivery environment, the positions and roles of those employed in the system as well as consumers will continue to change. Additionally, an emphasis on outcomes, both financial and clinical, are forcing professionals to examine patient and clinical data in innovative and resourceful ways. Incorporating the consumer of health care into the equation is probably the most dramatic change and emphasizes how information technology has promoted this shift.

CONSUMER PARTICIPATION IN HEALTH CARE

As information systems become more integrated and accessible via the WWW and consumers become more knowledgeable about health care, professionals will see a more informed and assertive public. The paradigm shift toward an emphasis on consumer informatics will alter the way health care professionals interact with patients and families. Supporting this shift are the latest statistics, which indicate that over 40% of American households have computers and 25% of all households have access to the Internet. From 1995 to 1999, there was an increase from 9% to 44% of people accessing the Internet from outside their homes. Access portals were located at work places, schools, community centers, and libraries (Department of Commerce, 1998). To date, there are over 25,000 health-related Internet sites and a majority of Internet users access health care information (Ferguson Report, 1999). A recent conference in New York brought together a coalition of consumers and health care providers to discuss topics ranging from health care research to consumer advocacy on the Internet (IHC '99). The increasing activism by consumers will mandate that professionals change the way they have been socialized in treating, teaching, and communicating with patients.

Armed with information obtained from digital consultants and networks, knowledgeable consumers are making decisions about their health care. In some instances, patients bypass the traditional system of health care providers and seek information based on personal choices alone and not necessarily scientific findings or prescriptive advice. However the information is obtained, patients are taking the initiative and making choices. Consumers are seeking data and information from peer groups; in other instances, sophisticated systems developed by professionals supply information based on patient preferences and sound clinical information (Brennan, 1998; Hovenga, Hovel, Klotz, & Robins, 1998; Ruland, 1999).

Nursing has traditionally considered patient values and beliefs in recommending care and treatment. The current emphasis on decision making supported by computer-mediated technology provides a new window in which to view and examine the process of decision making by consumers of health care. Much of the prior research reflected in the nursing literature on clinical decision making can be used to illuminate the area of clinical decision support and patient preferences currently under study in informatics.

Because automated programs are able to capture patient preferences and formulate appropriate decisions on a case-by-case basis, care can be customized and result in more effective and less expensive measures and strategies. (Balas, Boren, & Griffing, 1998; Brennan, et al., 1998; Ehnfors, Grobe, & Tallberg, 1998).

Finally, as nurses and other health care providers gradually incorporate patients into the health care process by the means of technology and telecommunications, the lack of access to digital systems by large segments of the population needs to be neutralized and corrected. Current statistics indicate that there is a "digital divide" among consumers of health care (Department of Commerce, 1998). Although access to computers and the Internet is becoming essential for both personal and economic success, major segments of our society do not have the ability or the means to become members of the digital society. The racial, economic, and educational disparity between the information "haves" and "have nots" continues to expand. Households with incomes of over $75,000 are 20 times more likely to have access to the Internet than those at the lower end of the economic strata; dual parent households are twice as likely to have Internet access than single-parent households, and the ownership disparity between whites, blacks, and Hispanics was greater in 1998 than 1995 (Department of Commerce, 1998). As advocates of patient care, health care professionals are in pivotal positions to support and promote access by all individuals regardless of economic and cultural class.

SUMMARY

We are experiencing sea changes in the financing, allocation, and process of health care. The explosion of a digital society has, to date, brought about transformations in the way people communicate, access, and process information. We are only beginning to understand the implications that the digital revolution will have on the way professionals practice, people change health practices, and health care is distributed and delivered. These are exciting times, but we will need a cadre of professionals who can think innovatively, practice in unconventional ways, and encourage empowered consumers to collaborate in their care. The education and practice systems will have to change to produce and support professionals in a dynamic, digital society. Research and development funds, both private and government, will play an important role in supporting an infrastructure that makes health education and care affordable, accessible, and effective. However, the educators and practitioners themselves will be the most important commodity in spearheading changes in their professions as well as in the health care delivery system of the future.

REFERENCES

American Nurses Association (1998). [On-Line] Available: *http://nursingworld.org/nidsec/index.htm.*

American Nurses Association (1994). *Scope of practice for nursing informatics.* Washington, DC: American Nurses Publishing.

AMIA Spring Conference (1999). Health Informatics Education. Chicago.

ANCC data on credential nurse practitioners. Telephone communication with Tina Todd of ANCC. September 10, 1999.

Arnold, J. (1996). Nursing informatics educational needs. *Computers in Nursing, 14* (6), 333–339.

Bakken, S., Cashen, M., & O'Brien, A. (1999). Evaluation of a type definition for representing nursing activities within a concept-based terminologic system. *Transforming Health Care through Informatics.* AMIA'99 Proceedings. CD-ROM.

Balas, E., Boren, S., & Griffing, G. (1998). Computerized management of diabetes: A synthesis of controlled trials. *A paradigm shift in health care information systems: Clinical infrastructures for the 21st century.* AMIA'98 Proceedings. CD-ROM.

Brennan, P. (1998). Improving health care by understanding patient preferences. (1998). *Journal of Medical Informatics Association, 5*(3), 257–262.

Brennan, P., Caldwell, B., Moore, S., Sreenath, N., & Jones, J. (1998). Designing heartcare: Custom computerized home care for patients recovering from CABG surgery. *A paradigm shift in health care information systems: Clinical infrastructures for the 21st century.* AMIA'98 Proceedings. CD-ROM.

Brennan, P., Moore, M., & Caldwell, B. (1999). Using WebTV to deliver information into the home: Experiences, successes and regrets. *Transforming Health Care through Informatics.* AMIA'99

Proceedings. CD-ROM.

Carty, B. (1994). The protean nature of the nurse informaticist. *Nursing and Health Care, 15*(4), 174–177.

Clark, D. (1997). The international classification for nursing practice: A progress report. In U. Gerdin, M. Tallberg, & P. Wainright (Eds.), *Nursing informatics: The impact of nursing knowledge on health care informatics* (pp. 62–68). Amsterdam: IOM Press.

CPRI (Computer-based Patient Record Institute). 1995 Guidelines for establishing Information Security Policies at Organizations Using Computer -Based Patient Record Systems. Schaumburg, Ill. CPRI

Corcoran-Perry S., & Graves, J. (1989). The study of nursing informatics. *Image Journal of Nursing Scholarship, 21*(4).

Department of Labor (1999). [On-Line] Available: URL: *www.dol.gov.*

Dick, R., Steen, E., & Detmer, D. (1997). The computer-based patient record. NAP. Washington, DC.

Ehnfors, M., Grobe, S., & Tallberg, M. (Eds.) (1998). *Nursing informatics: Combining clinical practice guidelines and patient preferences using health informatics.* SPRI, Stockholm.

Essex, D. (1999). Skip the song and dance. *Healthcare Informatics.* July, 1999.

Falling through the net II: New data on the digital divide (1998). [On-Line] Available: URL: *www.nita.doc.gov.*

Ferguson Report. (1999). [On-Line] Available: URL: *http://ferguson-report.sparklist.com.*

For the record: Protecting electronic health information (1997). The Committee on Maintaining Privacy and Security in Health Care Applications of the National Information Infrastructure, National Research Council. NAP, Washington, DC.

Gassert, C. (1998). The challenge of meeting patients' needs with a national nursing agenda. *Journal of Medical Informatics Association, 5*(3), 263–268.

Greenes, R., & Lorenzi, N. (1998). Audacious goals for health and biomedical informatics in the new millennium. *Journal of Medical Informatics Association, 5*(5), 395–400.

Grobe, S. J. (1996). The nursing intervention lexicon and taxonomy: Implications for representing nursing care data in automated records. *Holistic Nursing Practice, 11*(1), 48–63.

Henry, S., & Mead, C. (1997). Nursing classification systems: Necessary but not sufficient for representing "What Nurses Do." For inclusion in computer-based patient record systems. *Journal of Medical Informatics Association, 4*(3), 222–232.

Hovenga, E., Hovel, J., Klotz, J., & Robins, P. (1998). Infrastructure for reaching disadvantaged consumers: Telecommunications in rural and remote nursing in Australia. *Journal of Medical Informatics Association, 5*(3), 269–275.

Internet Healthcare Coalition (IHC). Proceedings: Quality healthcare information on the Net '99. New York, October 13, 1999. IHC.

Kelly, K. (1994). *Out of Control.* Addison-Wesley, New York.

Lang, N., Hudgings, C., Jacox, A., Lancour, J., McClure, M., McCormick, K., Saba, V., Stenvig, T., Zielstorff, R., Prescott, P., Milholland, D., O'Connor, K. (1995). Toward a national database for nursing practice. In N. Lang (Ed.), Nursing Data Systems: An Emerging Framework. Washington, DC: American Nurses Publishing.

Lindberg, C. (1997). Implementation of in-home telemedicine in rural Kansas: answering an elderly patient's needs. *Journal of Medical Informatics Association, 4*(1), 14–17.

Maas, M., Johnson, M., & Mooched, S. (1996). Classifying nursing-sensitive patient outcomes. *Image: Journal of Nursing Scholarship, 28*(4), 295–301.

McCormick, K. (1994). Toward standard classification schemes for nursing language: Recommendations of the American Nurses Association Steering Committee on databases to support clinical practice. *Journal of Medical Informatics Association, 1*(6), 421–427.

McGeady, Steven. (1999). The Internet as a Disruptive Force in Healthcare. *Healthcare Informatics.* July, 1999.

National Advisory Council on Nurse Education and Practice (1997). A National Informatics Agenda for Nursing Education. Department HRSA.

National Center Nursing Research (1993). *Nursing informatics: Enhancing patient care.* (NIH Publication No. 93–2419). Bethesda, MD: USA. National Center Nursing Research.

Patel, V., & Kaufman, D. (1998). Medical informatics and the science of cognition. *Journal of American Medical Informatics Association.* *5*(6), 493–501.

The registered nurse population. (1996). Findings from the National Sample Survey of Registered Nurses. U.S. Department of Health

& Human Services. HRSA. Bureau of Health Professions, Division of Nursing. Washington, DC.

Ribbons, R. (1998). The use of computers as cognitive tools to facilitate higher order thinking skills in nurse education. *Computers in Nursing, 16*(4), 223–228.

Ruland, C. (1999). Decision support for patient preference-based care planning: Effects on nursing care and patient outcomes. *Journal of Medical Informatics Association, 6*(4), 304–312.

Shortliffe E., & Greenes, R. (1990) Medical informatics: An emerging academic discipline and institutional discipline. *JAMA, 263*(8), 1114–1120.

Stead W. (1998). It's the information that's important, not the technology. *Journal of American Medical Informatics Association, 8*(1), 131.

Stead, W. (1999).The challenge to health informatics for 1999–2000: From creative partnerships with industry and chief information officers to enable people to use information to improve health. *Journal of Medical Informatics Association, 6*(1), 88–89.

Tang P., & Hammond, E. (1997). A progress report on computer-based patient records in the United States. In: *The Computer-Based Patient Record.* NAP. Washington, DC.

Tabar, P. (1999). The latest word. *Healthcare Informatics.* January, 1999.

The computer-based patient record: An essential technology for health care (1991). National Academy Press. Washington, DC.

Turley, J. (1996). Toward a model of nursing informatics. *Image: Journal of Nursing Scholarship, 28*(4), 309–313.

Zielstorff, R. (1997). A knowledge-based decision support system for the prevention and treatment of pressure ulcers. In U. Gerdin, M. Tallberg, P. Wainright, (Eds.), *Nursing informatics: The impact of nursing knowledge on health care informatics* (pp. 291–295). Amsterdam: IOM Press.

Zielstorff, R. (1995). Capturing and using clinical outcome data: implications for information systems design. *Journal of the Medical Informatics Association, 2*(3), 191–196.

Zielstorff, R., Tronni, C., Basgue, J., Griffin, L., Welebob, E., & Mapping, et al. (1998). Mapping nursing diagnosis nomenclatures for coordinated care. *Image: The Journal of Nursing Scholarship, 30*(4), 369–373.

2

Nursing Informatics: Competencies

Nancy Staggers and Carole Gassert

THE NEED FOR DEFINING NURSING INFORMATICS COMPETENCIES

In the midst of the information age, agreement does not exist about nurses' required competencies for information technology (IT) or informatics. The lack of such published work is a surprise given the pervasive amount of technology in nurses' work lives and the increasing use of the Internet by both nurses and patients. This chapter outlines work to date in defining Nursing Informatics (NI) competencies within the United States and, to a lesser extent, international organizations.

Despite the age of near ubiquitous computing, the integration of Nursing Informatics (NI) into nursing education in the United States has been sluggish. Johnson (1995) found that computer literacy was the only current health care emphasis not addressed by the majority of accredited baccalaureate nursing programs. A recent study of nursing programs showed little progress in that arena; less than one-third of the schools even addressed NI in their curricula (Carty & Rosenfeld, 1998).

Material is only beginning to appear about integrating NI into nursing curricula (Riley, 1996; Travis & Brennan, 1998; Vanderbeek & Beery, 1998). Travis and Brennan (1998) described an "innovative" curriculum to integrate NI into a baccalaureate nursing program. Riley (1996) outlined how computer technology is integrated into the baccalaureate program at Georgetown University. These kinds of descriptive articles can serve as essential guides for others; however, without agreement about competencies, each nursing program will define NI competencies and curricula uniquely.

U.S. national organizations have published only a few guidelines about information management and IT. For example, the American Association of Colleges of Nursing (AACN) (1998) provided seven broad guidelines related to information and health care technologies. Although the American Nurses Association (ANA) was a leader in defining the scope of practice for NI (ANA, 1994) and standards for the specialty (ANA, 1995), the organization has not yet published comprehensive material about NI competencies. In the international arena, the International Medical Informatics Association (IMIA) has drafted broad guidelines for competencies as well as informatics education (IMIA, 1999).

Defining specific informatics competencies is a crucial need. Gassert (1998) outlined national strategic directions for nursing, the result of recommendations from a panel of national NI experts in 1996. One of the foremost recommendations was to educate and prepare nursing students and practicing nurses in core NI competencies. The American Association of Colleges of Nursing (AACN) (1997) stated that within the next decade all nursing higher education must address priorities to include "the management of data and technology" (p. 2). The Pew Commission (Pew, 1998a) lists the effective and appropriate use of communication and information technologies as one of 21 essential competencies needed by all health professionals, including nursing, for the 21st century. In addition, the entire 1999 American Medical Informatics Association's (AMIA) Spring Congress was focused on education in health informatics. The conference emphasized the need for consensus on informatics competencies for all health disciplines.

Informatics competencies will be valuable to nursing for several reasons. The work on informatics competencies is foundational to determining educational needs for all nurses. Competencies are also useful for describing nurses' preparation in roles within practice, education, administration, and research (Grobe, 1989). Last, informatics competencies will be useful for developing nursing and health curricula, job descriptions, and managing the expectations of potential employers and consumers of health care.

Past Efforts in Defining NI Competencies

Despite the slow progress of integration into nursing, informatics competencies have been discussed since the early 1980s. In fact, over

36 articles were published on the topic. A number of authors outlined lists of various skills and knowledge nurses need (Armstrong, 1986; Bachman & Panzarine, 1998; Bryson, 1991; Carter & Axford, 1993; Walker & Walker, 1994). A frequently cited work to define nurses' informatics competencies was completed over 12 years ago by nursing members of the International Medical Informatics Association (Grobe, 1989; Peterson & Gerdin-Jelger, 1988). The task force defined three levels of competencies (user, developer, and expert) and developed informatics competencies according to these levels. Unfortunately, this work was never validated, and the competencies are now dated because they do not include contemporary advances in the field.

Across the 36 articles, authors did not agree upon needed informatics knowledge and skills. Many authors highlighted primarily technology skills (Armstrong, 1986; Carter & Axford, 1993; Saba & Riley, 1997; Walker & Walker, 1994). Except for Bryson (1991), authors seldom discussed the knowledge all nurses should have about informatics, such as privacy and confidentiality issues. The special skills nurse informaticists require, for example, techniques in systems analysis, system selection, and the evaluation of system impacts, are not emphasized. Informatics knowledge and skills for doctorally prepared informaticists were notably absent. More important, few articles addressed competencies for the range of nurses from baccalaureate to doctoral levels. With notable exceptions (Bachman & Panzarine 1998; Bryson, 1991; Carter & Axford, 1993), few of the articles reported empirically based recommendations.

A Definition of Nursing Informatics Competencies

The term competency is widely used in nursing education, administration, and practice without a precise understanding of its meaning. The general usage connotes a nuance of adequacy of behavior, but some authors equate the term skill with competency. Duffield (1989) even stated that competency and skills are interchangeable. Other authors disagreed, proposing that competency implies various attributes in addition to skills (Benner, 1982; Boss, 1985; May, Edell, Butell, Doughty, & Langford, 1999; McGee, Powell, Broadwell, & Clark, 1987; Nagelsmith, 1995). Thus, the concept of competency itself is a focus of conceptual confusion.

Authors offered a number of definitions for competency. Butler (1978, p. 7) defined competency as "the ability to meet or surpass prevailing standards of adequacy for a particular activity." Benner's (1984) seminal work was based upon competence as foundational to nursing. Nurses move through different levels of proficiency, including a middle level labeled "competent." At this level, nurses function capably with an increased capacity to assess situations globally, but they lack the versatility of experts. McGee et al. (1987) stated that competency meant the learned behaviors, knowledge, attitudes, and human traits specific to a given role. Mulholland (1994) defined the term as the ability to perform particular activities to a prescribed standard. Alspach (1992), on the other hand, separated the terms competence and competency; competence indicated the potential ability and capacity to function in a given situation while competency is based upon actual performance. Separating competence from competency is an interesting notion; however, it is confusing when made plural as both become the term "competencies."

Despite the array of definitions, authors agreed upon several issues: essential cognitive, psychomotor, and affective skills are needed, skill acquisition combines formal knowledge with experience, and competence implies an acceptable standard less than the expert level (May et al., 1999). Most authors think that competence is an integration of several abilities and that outcomes or performance measurement is necessary at some point to assess competence. Very consistently, authors define competency within a specific context or situation. Benner (1984) rightly acknowledged the difficulty of determining competencies, especially at the expert level. Determining standards for essential attributes like clinical judgment is exceptionally difficult. Even with that difficulty, the competency movement within nursing continues to grow. Therefore, a synthesis of ideas is offered in the following definition for NI competencies:

The integration of knowledge, skills, and attitudes in the performance of various NI activities within prescribed levels of nursing practice.

With a definition of NI competencies as a basis, the remaining sections of this chapter discuss guidelines and recommendations about informatics competencies from various organizations. The chapter concludes with specific NI competencies developed by an expert panel of national NI experts in conjunction with AMIA.

Pew Health Professions Commission (PHPC)

In 1998, the PHPC (Pew, 1998a) released its fourth and final report that focuses on health professions' education and practice. The report discusses nine trends that will shape health care and professional practice into the 21st century and recommends that health professions' education include a broader set of system, organizational, and population skills.

One of the trends discussed is the increasing use of information technology. PHPC states that increasingly health care providers must interact with patients who have obtained general health information or information about their disease state from the Internet. The report recognizes that in the future, all practitioners will need to be proficient in using information technologies to effectively manage the care of their patients.

In keeping with increased use of information technologies, PHPC has included the ability to use communication and IT as one of the essential competencies needed for practicing in the next century. Not only must nurses and other providers be able to use these technologies, they must use them effectively and appropriately in delivering care. PHPC recommends five activities that will assure student competence in using IT:

- Provide student access to electronic communication and information resources
- Structure learning assignments that require students to use electronic communication and information resources
- Provide learning experiences in clinical information management
- Incorporate educational technology in teaching-learning
- Develop partnerships with computer and software companies to develop and test the use of educational technologies and products.

American Association of Colleges of Nursing (AACN)

Recently, the AACN released a major revision to its document, "The Essentials of College and University Education for Professional Nursing" (AACN, 1998). A guide for nursing educational preparation into the 21st century, the document outlines core competencies for professional nursing education. The authors stated that technological advances will have a profound effect on disease prevention and detection, information management, and clinical decision making. More specifically, the document lists information and health care technologies as a core competency for nurses. According to the AACN, course work or clinical experiences should include the knowledge and skills to:

- Use information and communication technologies to document and evaluate patient care, advance patient education, and enhance the accessibility of care
- Use appropriate technologies in the process of assessing and monitoring patients
- Work in an interdisciplinary team to make ethical decisions regarding the application of technologies and the acquisition of data
- Adapt the use of technologies to meet patient needs
- Teach patients about health care technologies
- Protect the safety and privacy of patients in relation to the use of health care and information technologies, and
- Use information technologies to enhance one's own knowledge base (p. 9–10).

International Medical Informatics Association (IMIA)

IMIA (1999) published a draft document addressing international recommendations about education in Health and Medical Informatics. The recommendations focus on the knowledge and skills needed in information processing and IT for health care professionals as they progress in their careers and education. Learning outcomes are defined for two dimensions of professionals: IT users and informatics specialists. The document is based upon existing recommendations, primarily from European informaticists, and it provides generic recommendations for all health professionals, including nurses.

The full list of 41 recommendations is available at *www.imia.org/wg1* and is further annotated by three levels of complexity titled introductory, principles and profound knowledge/skills. Sample recommendations from the section on processing data, information, and knowledge include:

- Benefits and current constraints of using IT in health care
- General principles of health information systems
- Construction of health coding systems and their representation principles
- Appropriate decision making, using and constructing guidelines and critical paths

The methods and technology section includes:

- Data analysis
- Medical image processing, and
- Ethical issues pertaining to confidentiality, privacy and security of patient data.

Among others, the organizational section includes:

- Fundamentals of human functioning
- Organization of the health system, and
- Health administration, health economics, health quality and resource management, public health services and outcome measurement.

The fourth section on informatics/computer science section includes:

- Basic informatics terms,
- Using personal computers,
- Change management and project management,
- Mathematics, and biometry.

IMIA further divides this varied list into two specializations—an informatics-based approach to health and medical informatics and a health care–based approach. The first emphasizes profound knowledge and skills of health informatics, mathematics, and computer science. In the second, health education is a primary focus with informatics as a support. IMIA outlines sample course recommendations from baccalaureate to doctoral levels. IMIA is currently soliciting comments about its document and submitted recommendations to the IMIA general assembly for approval in November, 1999.

The IMIA document is an important contribution in the move toward worldwide standardization of health informatics curricula. It is a generic guide to overall concepts for education and a contrast to the effort in AMIA, discussed later in this chapter, which outlines more specific competencies for nurses. Both perspectives are valuable as underpinnings for the future.

Nursing Informatics Standards and Certification

As indicated earlier, the ANA published the scope of practice and standards document for nursing informatics practice (ANA, 1994, 1995). Two different panels of informatics experts produced the documents. In describing what NI is and is not, the scope of practice document identifies two levels of informatics practice for nurses. The informatics nurse is described as one who has a bachelor's degree in nursing and additional knowledge and experience in the field of informatics. Twelve competencies are listed as requisite for this level of practice. The competencies, however, are listed primarily as topics and not as competency statements. Six of the topics relate to the systems development life cycle. Additional topics include networks, human computer interface, translator skills, and use of principles from other disciplines.

The second level of informatics practice described in the ANA document is the informatics nurse specialist (INS). This nurse must have a master's degree in nursing and have taken graduate-level courses in informatics. The document states the INS must be competent in seven areas. Four of these areas relate to the systems development life cycle. Other areas include developing and teaching theory and practice of NI, consultation practice in NI, and collaboration with other health informatics specialists. Although statements about the INS's practice are more specific in terms of behavior, the document lacks sufficient detail to judge the competence of an INS's practice.

The ANA (1995) document states that it delineates standards of practice for the specialty of NI. According to the document itself, however, it "describes a generalist level of nursing informatics practice..." (p. 1). The generalist level corresponds to the informatics nurse described in the previous scope of practice document. Standards for the INS level of practice, the graduate nurse with additional preparation in informatics, are not included.

By listing both practice standards and professional standards, the NI standards document follows a format commonly used by ANA. Not surprisingly, practice standards for the informatics nurse include assessment, diagnosis, outcome identification, planning, implementation, and evaluation activities. Professional standards address quality, performance appraisal, education, collegiality, ethics, collaboration, research, and resource utilization in informatics. In a third section, the document identifies informatics domain standards for the IN. The five categories of domain standards are information systems life cycle, principles and theories, information technology, communication, and databases.

Standards are considered to be "authoritative statements in which the nursing profession describes the responsibilities for which nurses are accountable" (ANA, 1995, p. 1). The NI standards document has produced statements that can be used to evaluate the practice of the informatics nurse, the generalist in nursing informatics. It has also been used as a basis for certification in NI.

Nursing Informatics Certification.

A certification examination for credentialing nurses as generalists in NI was developed by the ANA, through its affiliate, the American Nurses Credentialing Center (ANCC) in 1995. The certification examination test content outline is as follows:

- System analysis and design
- System implementation and support
- System testing and evaluation
- Human factors
- Computer technology
- Information/database management
- Professional practice trends and issues
- Theories

The certification examination is computer-based and available on demand. To be eligible to sit for the examination, nurses must be currently licensed in the United States, hold a baccalaureate or higher degree, and have practiced a minimum of two years as a nurse. In addition, the nurse must have either 2000 hours of practice in the field of informatics nursing within the past 5 years or have completed 12 semester hours of informatics in a graduate program and practiced 1000 hours in informatics nursing within the past 5 years (ANCC, 1999a). Since the NI certification examination was first administered in 1995, more than 97% of examinees have passed and become certified as informatics nurses (ANCC, 1999b). The passing rate for informatics nurses is much higher than the passing rate for most of the other generalist tests, including the basic registered nurse exam.

The NI community has benefited significantly from the existence of certification, one of the five requirements for an area of practice to be considered a specialty in nursing. As indicated, however, certification for informatics nurse specialists prepared at the master's level is lacking. Master's prepared nurses who practice in informatics must take a generalist examination if they wish to become certified in informatics, a fact that may inflate the passing rate for the informatics certification examination. Furthermore, standards of practice for the INS have not been sufficiently delineated to reflect this more advanced level of informatics practice. As technology becomes more complex, and more ubiquitous, the NI community may benefit from the differentiation of levels of practice in NI, including the doctoral level.

Continued Competency

The PHPC (October, 1998b) indicated that health care workforce regulation must focus on three areas to achieve greater consumer protection: health professions boards and governance structures, scope of practice authority, and continued competence. In addressing continued competence, the PHPC states that state regulatory boards should expand their responsibilities beyond individuals entering professional practice and require all practitioners to demonstrate competence throughout their professional career.

Licensing examinations administered by state boards of nursing are designed to assure a minimal level of competence in nursing practice. Demonstration of continued competence is not generally required of nurses. Some state boards require evidence of continuing education, but these requirements do not assure continued competence. Some in nursing advocate periodic re-examination for re-licensure in nursing. Others feel that testing only measures knowledge, not competence (ANA, 1999). The ANA, National Council of State Boards of Nursing, specialty organizations, and other professional organizations are currently focusing on how to assure continued competence. If the field of NI is to assure that its practitioners are competent, differentiating between basic and more advanced informatics competencies is imperative.

American Medical Informatics Association (AMIA)—NI Expert Panel:

The University of Utah identified the need for explicating specific NI competencies to guide the integration of informatics throughout the entire nursing curricula. Dr. Gassert began similar work while at the University of Maryland. These two efforts were combined and expanded. To begin, initial informatics competencies for nurses were abstracted from 35 articles and 14 job descriptions from practicing nurse informaticists. The resulting list included 1,159 items. These initial competencies were reviewed by the two NI experts and classified into inductively derived categories for consolidation. For example, one competency was "Employ an authoring language to develop computer-assisted instruction." This item was labeled Computer Assisted Instruction (CAI). After all items were similarly categorized, the categories were then used to sort initial competencies in a database and eliminate redundant items. The resulting list included 313 unique items after consolidation.

An expert panel with national representation was then convened in December, 1998, to develop and refine these NI competencies. Members included doctorally prepared NI representatives from academe and industry at NYU (Barbara Carty, EdD, RN); the Division of Nursing, Department of Health and Human Services (Carole Gassert, PhD, RN); PennState Health Systems (Christine Curran, PhD, RN, University of Maryland); Syracuse University (Ramona Nelson, PhD, RN); and the University of Utah (Rita Snyder-Halpern, PhD, RN and Nancy Staggers, PhD, RN, FAAN). Drs. Staggers and Gassert led the development effort and coordinated it with the AMIA Nursing Informatics Working Group.

The expert panel began validating the 313 competencies; however, the members quickly discovered that they were unable to progress without defining a nursing context for the competencies. Therefore, the group defined four levels of nurses: beginning, experienced, informatics specialist, and informatics innovator. Definitions were created for these nurse levels. To begin consensus about competencies by nurse level, each panel member separately rated all competencies. An 80% level was established as the threshold for agreement about an item. Items outside that range were discussed and either clarified and leveled or eliminated. Only a few competencies were eliminated because they were clearly outdated, for example, skills in using a fax machine. Several others that were eliminated did not address competencies specific to informatics but were generic to nursing, for example, "Practices according to the Code for Nurses."

After leveling, the panel noted that the informatics innovator category was underdeveloped. Competencies were created to describe the doctorally prepared informatics innovator. Additionally, the panel reworded competencies across levels to reflect the increases in complexity from beginner to innovator. Bloom's taxonomy (cited in Waltz, Strickland, & Lenz, 1991) was used to determine appropriate verbs for each level. A sample list of the competencies created by the expert panel is listed in Appendix A. This work is summarized in Staggers, Gassert, and Curran (in press).

The next step in validating these NI competencies is to conduct a larger study using a Delphi technique in a sample of NI nurses. Funding for the effort was obtained from the University of Utah College of Nursing. The projected completion date for the project is late fall, 2000. Further information about this study and its results are available from the authors.

SUMMARY

The need for determining Nursing Informatics competencies is clear. National organizations such as the AACN and Pew Commission have recommended that IT and informatics be included in health curricula. The work about competencies discussed here can serve as the underpinnings to defining standardized NI curricula.

Multiple efforts are now underway to define informatics competencies including those in AMIA and IMIA. IMIA defined broad guidelines about informatics education for health professionals and informaticists. These guidelines will need to be more defined more specifically before being implemented, however. The specific competencies outlined by the NI expert panel in AMIA resulted in a master list of 304 NI skills and knowledge areas across 4 levels of NI practice. This effort provides a research-based approach to defining NI competencies. While agreement about the specifics of NI competencies across organizations does not yet exist, the broad guidelines of IMIA and specific competencies in AMIA are complementary efforts and have the promise of convergence in the future.

Once consensus about required competencies is achieved, a core set can be determined. Likewise, a phased approach to career-long education and mastery of extensive competencies can be outlined. One method of managing the broad base of entry-level NI competencies and the rapid change in this field may be to require nurses to develop a portfolio to track their own NI skills and knowledge. Based upon standards and validated NI competencies, tracking competencies in this manner would also be useful as organizations move toward continuing competence.

Further work in competencies is needed to compare and contrast defined levels of professionals, knowledge domains, skills, and delineated foci of programs for health professionals. Differentiating NI practice levels is also imperative for the near future to define competencies, credentialing, and continued competence for the master's and doctorally prepared nurse informaticist.

In the age of near ubiquitous computing, nursing informatics competencies will be as basic to nursing education and continued competence as performing a health history is today. Over the next five years, expect NI competencies to be defined and accepted and vast improvement in the numbers of nursing programs including NI in their curricula at all levels of training. On the individual level, nurses can take personal responsibility in the managing their own NI education by creating and tracking their portfolio of NI competencies.

APPENDIX I
SAMPLE NURSING INFORMATICS COMPETENCIES
NI EXPERT PANEL

SAMPLE NURSING INFORMATICS COMPETENCIES

Level 1 Beginning Nurse

1. Uses administrative applications for practice management (e.g., searches for patient, retrieves demographics, billing data)
2. Uses telecommunication devices (e.g., modems or other devices) to communicate with other systems (e.g., access data, upload, download)
3. Uses e-mail (e.g., create, send, respond, use attachments)
4. Uses the Internet to locate, download items of interest (e.g., patient, nursing resources)
5. Uses a database management program to develop a simple database and/or table
6. Identifies the appropriate technology to capture the required patient data (e.g., fetal monitoring device)
7. Seeks available resources to help formulate ethical decisions in computing

Level 2 Experienced Nurse

1. Uses applications for diagnostic coding
2. Evaluates CAI as a teaching tool
3. Extracts selected literature resources and integrates them to a personally usable file
4. Supports efforts toward development and use of a unified nursing language
5. Defines the impact of computerized information management on the role of the nurse
6. Assesses the accuracy of health information on the Internet
7. Acts as an advocate of system users including patients or clients

Level 3 Informatics Specialist

1. Has the ability to integrate different applications or programs
2. Constructs guidelines for the purchase of software and hardware
3. Determines projected impacts to users and organizations when changing to computerized information management
4. Analyzes business practices to determine need for reengineering
5. Prepares process flow charts to describe current and proposed information flows for all aspects of clinical systems
6. Develops screen layouts, report formats, and custom views of clinical data working directly with clinical departments and individual users
7. Devises strategies for installing applications/systems

Level 4 Informatics Innovator

1. Designs innovative analytic techniques
2. Designs unique technology or system alternatives for clinical care, education, administration, and/or research
3. Develops the conceptual model for a database
4. Evaluates factors related to safety, effectiveness, cost, and social impact when developing and implementing information management technologies
5. Develops strategies to obtain research funding
6. Conducts basic science research to support the theoretical development of the informatics specialty (e.g., decision making, human-computer interaction, taxonomy development, etc.)
7. Applies advanced methodological and statistical techniques to the design and evaluation of computerized clinical information systems

REFERENCES

AACN (1997). *A vision of baccalaureate and graduate nursing education: The next decade.* Washington, D.C.: American Association of Colleges of Nursing.

AACN (1998). *Essentials of baccalaureate education for professional nursing practice.* Washington, D.C.: American Association of Colleges of Nursing.

Alspach, G. (1992). Concern and confusion over competence [editorial]. *Critical Care Nurse, 12*(4), 9–11.

American Nurses Association (1994). *The scope of practice for nursing informatics.* Washington, D.C.: American Nurses Publishing.

American Nurses Association (1995). *Standards of practice for nursing informatics.* Washington, D.C.: American Nurses Publishing.

American Nurses Association (1999). Should registered nurses have to periodically take an exam to be relicensed as proof of their continued competence? [On-Line] Available: *http://www.nursingworld.org/tan/99janfeb/kaleid.htm.*

American Nurses Credentialing Center (1999a). ANCC Informatics Nurse Certification Catalog. [On-Line] Available: *http://www.ana.org/ancc/certify/catalogs/1998/inform98/infomat.htm.*

American Nurses Credentialing Center (1999b). Certification Exam Results. [On-Line]. Available: *http://www.ana.org/acnn/exams.htm.*

Armstrong, M. L. (1986). Computer competence for nurse educators. *Image: Journal of Nursing Scholarship, 18*(4), 155–60.

Bachman, J. A., & Panzarine, S. (1998). Enabling student nurses to use the information superhighway. *Journal of Nursing Education, 37*(4), 155–61.

Benner, P. (1982). Issues in competency-based testing. *Nursing Outlook, 30*(5), 303–9.

Benner, P. (1984). *From novice to expert: Excellence and power in clinical nursing practice.* Menlo Park, CA: Addison-Wesley.

Boss, L. A. (1985). Teaching for clinical competence. *Nurse Educator, 10*(4), 8–12.

Bryson, D. M. (1991). The computer-literate nurse. *Computers in Nursing, 9*(3), 100–7.

Butler, F. C. (1978). The concept of competence: An operational definition. *Educational Technology, 7*, 7–18.

Carter, B. E., & Axford, R. L. (1993). Assessment of computer learning needs and priorities of registered nurses practicing in hospitals. *Computers in Nursing, 11*(3), 122–6.

Carty, B., & Rosenfeld, P. (1998). From computer technology to information technology. Findings from a national study of nursing education. *Computers in Nursing, 16*(5), 259–65.

Duffield, C. (1989). The competencies expected of first-line nursing managers—an Australian context. *Journal of Advanced Nursing, 14*(12), 997–1001.

Gassert, C. A. (1998). The challenge of meetings patients' needs with a national nursing informatics agenda. *Journal of the American Medical Informatics Association, 5*(3), 263–268.

Grobe, S. J. (1989). Nursing informatics competencies. *Methods of Information in Medicine, 28*(4), 267–9.

IMIA (1999). *Recommendations of the International Medical Informatics Association (IMIA) on education in health and medical informatics.* (Draft): International Medical Informatics Association. Available: *http://www. imia.org/wg1.*

Johnson, J. Y. (1995). Curricular trends in accredited generic baccalaureate nursing programs across the United States. *Journal of Nursing Education, 34*(2), 53–60.

May, B. A., Edell, V., Butell, S., Doughty, J., & Langford, C. (1999). Critical thinking and clinical competence: a study of their relationship in BSN seniors [see comments]. *Journal of Nursing Education, 38*(3), 100–110.

McGee, R. F., Powell, M. L., Broadwell, D. C., & Clark, J. C. (1987). A Delphi survey of oncology clinical nurse specialist competencies. *Oncology Nurse Forum, 14*(2), 29–34.

Mulholland, J. (1994). Competency-based learning applied to nursing management. *Journal of Nursing Management, 2*(4), 161–6.

Nagelsmith, L. (1995). Competence: an evolving concept. *Journal of Continuing Education in Nursing, 26*(6), 245–8.

Peterson, H., & Gerdin-Jelger, V. (1988). *Preparing nurses for using information systems: Recommended informatics competencies.* New York: NLN Publications.

Pew Health Professions Commission (1998a). Recreating health professional practice for a new century: The fourth report of the Pew Health Professions Commission. San Francisco, CA: Pew Health Professions Commission.

Pew Health Professions Commission (1998b). Strengthening consumer protection: Priorities for health care workforce regulation. San Francisco, CA: Pew Health Professions Commission.

Riley, J. B. (1996). Educational applications. In V. K. Saba & K. A. McCormick (Eds.), *Essentials of computers for nurses* (2nd ed.). New York: McGraw Hill.

Saba, V. K., & Riley, J. B. (1997). Nursing informatics in nursing education. *Studies in Health Technology and Informatics, 46,* 185–90.

Staggers, N. Gassert, C. & Curran, C. (In press). Informatics at four levels of practice. Journal of Nursing Education.

Travis, L., & Flatley-Brennan, P. (1998). Information science for the future: an innovative nursing informatics curriculum. *Journal of Nursing Education, 37*(4), 162–8.

Vanderbeek, J., & Beery, T. A. (1998). A blueprint for an undergraduate healthcare informatics course. *Nurse Educator, 23*(1), 15–9.

Walker, P. H., & Walker, J. M. (1994). Informatics for nurse managers: integrating clinical expertise, business applications, and technology. *Seminars for Nurse Managers, 2*(2), 63–71.

Waltz, C., Strickland, O. & Lenz. E. (1991). Measurement in nursing research (2nd Ed.). NY: F. A. Davis.

3

Core Informatics: Content for an Undergraduate Curriculum

Ramona Nelson

The focus of this chapter is the integration of core nursing informatics concepts in the undergraduate curriculum. The chapter is written as a resource for faculty and administrators responsible for planning, implementing, and evaluating undergraduate nursing curriculum. This includes programs offering an associate degree, a diploma, and/or a baccalaureate degree. Graduates from these programs use automated patient care systems to manage and document patient care. This chapter provides resources and suggested content that can be used in preparing graduates for these important roles.

CONTENT BASE FOR TEACHING INFORMATICS

The first undergraduate nursing course focused on computer technology was offered at the State University of New York at Buffalo in 1977 (Saba & McCormick, 1995). Over the last 20 years, an increasing number of undergraduate programs have introduced courses dealing with computers in health care or nursing informatics. The process for introducing these courses has followed a haphazard pattern. Initially, many courses were established as electives by faculty who had developed a personal interest in computers. A major resource for planning these courses was a small book by Judith Ronald and Diane Skiba (Ronald & Skiba, 1987). This reference, written as a guide for faculty, included both computer literacy and nursing informatics content.

Many of the initial courses focused on PC-based computer literacy with limited information related to nursing informatics. Often the course content was not used or referred to in any other nursing courses. Three major forces have changed that picture. First, health care delivery is increasingly dependent on automation and faculty are much more aware of this impact. Second, with the advent of the Internet, computer use is becoming a part of everyday life for all citizens. Third, both students and faculty are increasingly computer literate.

Today, the inclusion of health care or nursing informatics content in the undergraduate curriculum follows the same systematic process used for all curriculum revisions and updates. This includes assessment of the informatics-related learning needs, planning of the curriculum, implementing the learning experiences, and evaluating the learning outcomes. The assessment process is used to identify program, year, and level objectives as well as the appropriate content to be included in each level of the curriculum. Curriculum planning for nursing informatics begins with the assessment of three content areas. These content areas are computer literacy, information literacy, and nursing informatics. These areas of content are presented in Figure 3.1.

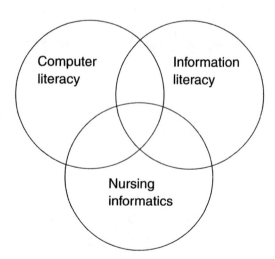

FIGURE 3.1 Relationships and interrelationships of computer literacy, information literacy and nursing informatics.

As can be seen in Figure 3.1, each of these subjects includes content that is independent of the others as well as content that overlaps. When planning the curriculum it is important to identify the content within each of these areas as well as the overlap and interrelationships between these areas of content. Because computer literacy and information literacy are prerequisite for understanding nursing informatics, course content related to these topics should occur early in the nursing program, usually in the freshman year or beginning of the sophomore year.

Nursing informatics focuses on using automation to manage nursing information. This content can be integrated throughout the curriculum; however, students need a basic understanding of nursing information and health care delivery before they can comprehend nursing informatics. For example, students will not understand issues related to automated charting if they have never been introduced to the nursing process and the use of standard languages.

COMPUTER LITERACY

Computer Literacy is defined as a knowledge of computers combined with the ability to use them effectively. ("Computer Literacy," 1993–1996). This definition suggests that planning for computer literacy within a nursing curriculum begins with the faculty discussing the level and type of computer literacy required of a professional nurse. In discussing this question there are three issues faculty need to consider. These are:

1. What computer literacy–related program, year, or level goals should be established? What learning experiences and content should be included in the undergraduate nursing curriculum so that students can achieve the identified goals?
2. Should computer literacy be taught by nursing faculty or other university faculty?
3. How should nursing students learn to integrate computer literacy concepts into their role as health care providers?

These issues can be explored by analyzing Figure 3.2.

The circle represents computer literacy. Overlapping this circle is information literacy and nursing informatics. The area of Figure 3.2

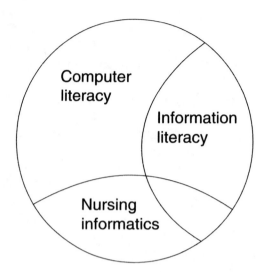

FIGURE 3.2 The overlap of information literacy and nursing informatics with computer literacy.

that does not overlap with information literacy or nursing informatics represents computer literacy knowledge and skills that can be expected of all graduates irrespectful of major. The overlap with information literacy is the level of computer literacy needed to access, evaluate, and use automated information resources. The overlap with nursing informatics represents specific computer literacy skills needed to use computers in delivering health care.

Establishing Computer Literacy Goals and Content

There are several resources that faculty can use to identify computer literacy goals and content for the undergraduate nursing curriculum. The assessment process includes both an internal scan and an external scan. The external scan examines computer literacy influences outside of the university. The internal scan evaluates what is happening across the university as a whole as well as within departments and schools.

It is often helpful to begin with an internal scan. Many universities have established or are in the process of establishing computer literacy outcomes or goals that apply to all graduates. Ideally, faculty representatives from the school/department of nursing are working with other college or university faculty to establish the level of computer literacy expected of all graduates. In addition, many university departments and programs are in the process of establishing computer literacy outcomes. The goals and outcome measures developed by these faculty colleagues can be important resources for nursing faculty. Virginia Commonwealth University provides an example of a university establishing computer literacy goals. Their report can be seen at *http://www.vcu.edu/provost/restructuring978/technologycompetency.html* ("Technology Competency of Graduates in Virginia Commonwealth University's," 1998).

Another resource for establishing goals and evaluating potential course content includes computer literacy courses developed by faculty colleagues in other departments. Examples can be found externally on the Internet as well as internally on the local campus. Some common course titles include *Computer Applications, Introduction to Computers* and *Computer Concepts.* Using these terms with a general search engine produces several examples of computer literacy courses on the Internet. A major resource for finding courses on the Internet is the World Lecture Hall located at *http://www.utexas.edu/world/lecture/.*

Faculty should look for examples of course syllabi that include computer lab experiences and homework assignments with a variety of software packages. Computer literacy is a cognitive and psychomotor skill. Students need an opportunity to practice. Table 3.1 lists the content topics and examples of the software that are often used to teach computer literacy.

Reviewing courses on the Internet is the beginning of the external scan. The external scan also includes an analysis of high school requirements. A major resource in conducting this aspect of the assessment is the United States Department of Education.

One of the first major educational reports that included computer literacy was *A Nation At Risk* by the National Commission on Excellence in Education (1983). As early as 1983, the commission recommended that all students take one-half year of computer science. This report and a number of follow-up reports and statistics can be accessed at the Department of Education's web site at *http://www.ed.gov/.*

Computer technology and software changes rapidly. As a result,

TABLE 3.1 Basic Computer Literacy Content

Content	Examples
Underlying concepts	
Hardware including peripherals	CPU, printer, modem
Operating system	Windows 2000, Unix, Macintosh
Productivity software	
Word Processing	WordPerfect(r)
	Microsoft Word
Spreadsheet software	Quattro(r) Pro
	Microsoft Excel
Database software	Paradox(r)
	Microsoft Access
Graphics	Corel(r) Presentations'
	Microsoft PowerPoint
Common applications	
Desktop publishing	Adobe PageMaker
Personal information manager	Corel(r) InfoCentral'
Statistics	SPSS, Minitab

computer literacy objectives, goals, and content often need to be reviewed and revised on a yearly basis.

Identifying faculty to teach computer literacy

The second issue is, should basic computer literacy content be taught by nursing faculty? The answer is—that depends. The definition of computer literacy includes the phase "the ability to use them effectively." For health care providers, computer literacy includes the ability to use computers effectively in health care. To use computers effectively in health care, nursing students need to have mastered basic computer literacy. These are the same computer literacy skills all students need to master. However, they also need to learn how to apply these skills in managing nursing information. For example, nursing students should be able to use a word processing or desktop publishing program to create a teaching booklet for a group of patients. The students should be able to create the booklet, measure the reading level when the booklet content includes medical terminology, and make appropriate modifications to be sure patients are able to understand and use the booklet.

If there are computer literacy course(s) offered on campus that meet the general computer literacy goals of the nursing curriculum, these courses can be included the nursing curriculum. With this approach, nursing courses are reviewed for computer-related content to ensure that nursing students learn to apply computer skills within their profession. The other approach is to include general computer literacy within nursing courses. A reference that can be used with either approach is *Computers in Small Bytes* (Joos, Whitman, Smith, & Nelson, 2000). This is a computer literacy book for health care professionals with several activities designed to aid nursing students in developing computer skills using health care information.

As noted in Figure 3.2, computer literacy skills overlap with information literacy skills. Table 3.2 includes a list of skills that fall within this area. These are basic computer literacy skills that are necessary for information literacy.

INFORMATION LITERACY

Information literacy skills can be grouped into three areas. These are the ability to effectively and efficiently access information, evaluate accessed information, and determine appropriate uses of information. Information literacy overlaps with nursing informatics when the information being accessed, evaluated, and utilized is health-related information. Because information literacy is a basic skill required by all programs of higher education, faculty should use the same approach for identifying outcomes and skills that are recommended for identifying basic computer literacy. That is, work within the university structure to develop outcomes and learning experiences that apply to all students. In addition, nursing students need to apply information literacy skills to health-related information. For example, all students should know how to do an on-line literature search. However, nursing students need to know the difference between CINAHL and MEDLINE.

TABLE 3.2 Overlaping Computer Literacy And Information Literacy Skills

Content	Examples
Establishing connections	
Connecting to a local area network	
Connecting to the Internet	
Communication skills	
E-mail	
Discussion boards	
Listservers	
Newgroups	
Chat	
Information access skills	
Basic concepts	Using a browser
	Boolean search strategies
Search engines	Yahoo
	Altavista
Common applications	
Creating Web pages	Adobe PageMaker
Web-based distance education software	

Resources for Establishing Information Literacy Objectives and Goals

University librarians and professional library organizations are primary resources for curriculum planning related to information literacy for all students. Faculty planning information literacy–related curriculum content are encouraged to make an appointment with the appropriate reference librarian early in the curriculum planning process. Table 3.3 includes standards of information literacy that have been published by the American Library Association.

TABLE 3.3 Information Power

The Nine Information Literacy Standards For Student Learning

Excerpted from Chapter 2, "Information Literacy Standards for Student Learning," of Information Power: Building Partnerships for Learning. Copyright© 1998 American Library Association and Association for Educational Communications and Technology.

Information Literacy

Standard 1: The student who is information literate accesses information efficiently and effectively.

Standard 2: The student who is information literate evaluates information critically and competently.

Standard 3: The student who is information literate uses information accurately and creatively.

Independent Learning

Standard 4: The student who is an independent learner is information literate and pursues information related to personal interests.

Standard 5: The student who is an independent learner is information literate and appreciates literature and other creative expressions of information.

Standard 6: The student who is an independent learner is information literate and strives for excellence in information seeking and knowledge generation.

Social Responsibility

Standard 7: The student who contributes positively to the learning community and to society is information literate and recognizes the importance of information to a democratic society.

Standard 8: The student who contributes positively to the learning community and to society is information literate and practices ethical behavior in regard to information and information technology.

Standard 9: The student who contributes positively to the learning community and to society is information literate and participates effectively in groups to pursue and generate information.

Copyright © 1999, American Library Association. Last Modified: Monday, 16-Nov-1998 15:54:58 CST

The URL of the homepage for the American Library Association is located at *http://www.ala.org*. The information literacy standards can be accessed at *http://www.ala.org/aasl/ip_nine.html*. One of the units within the American Library Association is the Association of College & Research Libraries. The web page for this unit is located at *http://www.ala.org/acrl/*. This unit is developing *Information Literacy Competency Standards for Higher Education*. The standards and performance indicators included in this document are especially useful to nursing faculty developing curriculum objectives and educational outcomes for an undergraduate nursing curriculum.

Information literacy includes the ability to access and use both automated and nonautomated information resources. However the focus in this chapter is on automated information resources where information literacy overlaps with computer literacy and nursing informatics. What do nursing students need to understand in order to access, evaluate, and use information stored in automated databases and accessed via a computer?

Prerequisite Knowledge for Information Literacy

Many people manage to access information using library databases and the Internet without understanding the databases that they are searching or the searching tools that they are using. For example, many people know how to start a search engine, insert a word or phrase, click on go, and look at the results. The results from this type of a search have two major deficits. First, they lack specificity. Many of the URLs and documents in the results are irrelevant. Second, the results lack sensitivity. There are many key URLs or documents that are missing or so far down the long list of results that the user never sees them. Information literacy is the ability to effectively and efficiently access information with sensitivity and specificity.

An understanding of three basic concepts underlies using effective and efficient strategies for accessing information. These concepts apply when students are searching the Internet, literature databases, or health care information systems. Information is stored in databases. An understanding of database structure is the first concept. Data stored in a database are indexed. If the index or standard language that was established when the database was developed is used to search that database the results are much more specific. For example, searching a literature database such as MEDLINE with the subject words that were used to index MEDLINE produces results that are much more specific and sensitive to the search question. Searching with key words is the same as doing a string search. The results are less sensitive and specific.

The second concept is the difference between a database and database management system. For example, an Internet search engine is a database management system while the Internet is the database. MEDLINE is a literature database that can be searched using many different database management systems. The university library may be offering access to MEDLINE using a commercial database management system. Students searching MEDLINE using PubMed from the NLM are using a different database management system to search this same database. Different results may be obtained with these two approaches to searching MEDLINE because the database management systems are different. This same concept applies to the healthcare information systems and searching for patient data.

The third concept involves Boolean search strategies. Boolean search strategies are used to expand a search (increased sensitivity) or limit a search (increased specificity). The most common Boolean search strategies involve the use of AND, OR and NOT. AND expands a search, while OR, and NOT limits a search.

Resources for Teaching Students to Access Information

Most university libraries provide classes and handouts for orienting students to the library and the resources in the library. For nursing students this orientation should include the literature databases that are specific to health care. Some important examples are MEDLINE, CINAHL, and HealthStar.

In addition, students use the Internet and a variety of search engines available on the Internet. Table 3.4 includes a number of web-based resources that can be used to teach about search engines including those that are specific to health care.

Resources for Teaching Students to Evaluate Information

Previous to the Internet, nursing students usually searched for information in professional books and journals that had been carefully reviewed and edited. The quality of the information was not usually

TABLE 3.4 Web Resources Useful in Teaching Information Access

URL	Title and Author
http://tlc.nlm.nih.gov/resources/tutorials/ healthsciencedistancelearning/ coverpage.html	Health science distance learning Applications on the Internet by Michael Weisberg, EdD and Craig Locatis, PhD
http://www.web-action.com/search-engines/index.html	Understanding search engines
http://www.nursing.uconn.edu/cybrtour.html	The cybertourtorials: Historical online readings by Susan Sparks
http://www.nnlm.nlm.nih.gov/tools.html	Internet discovery tools: Guides to health resources maintained by National Library of Medicine.
http://axe.uoregon.edu/network/learn-search-engines.html	Learn more about search engines maintained by the University of Oregon Library System
http://www.angelfire.com/in/virtuallibrarian/ index.html	The cyberlibrarians' rest stop

a concern. Today, many students start with the Internet and if not encouraged to use other resources will limit their efforts to this resource. On the Internet they often find the latest and best information mixed with outdated, inaccurate, and misleading information. A number of university libraries and others have developed resources that can be used in teaching students how to evaluate the quality of information. Many of these resources focus on applying information literacy skills to materials posted on the Internet. Table 3.5 includes a list of web sites that can be used for this purpose.

TABLE 3.5 Web Resources Useful in Teaching Evaluation of Information

URL	Title and Author
http://www2.widener.edu/Wolfgram-Memorial-Library/webeval.htm	Evaluating web resources by Jan Alexander and Marsha Ann Tate
http://www.ala.org/parentspage/greatsites/criteria.html	Selection criteria: How to tell if you are looking at a great web site by ALSC Children and Technology Committee.
http://sosig.ac.uk/desire/internet-detective.html	Internet detective owner, DESIRE, contact: desire-demo@bris.ac.uk
http://itech1.coe.uga.edu/Faculty/GWilkinson/criteria.html	Evaluating the quality of Internet information sources: Consolidated listing of evaluation criteria and quality indicators by Gene L. Wilkinson, Lisa T. Bennett, and Kevin M. Oliver
http://milton.mse.jhu.edu:8001/research/education/net.html	Evaluating information found on the Internet by Elizabeth E. Kirk
http://www.vuw.ac.nz/~agsmith/evaln/evaln.htm	Evaluation of information sources by Alastair Smith

Resources for Teaching About Health-Related Information Literacy.

Just as undergraduate nursing students should become cognizant of nursing and health care literature, they also need to become familiar with resources for ensuring access to quality health care information on the Internet. With the advent of the Internet, many clients are using the same information resources that professionals are using. Both healthcare professionals and clients are accessing quality health-related information mixed with inaccurate and misleading information. Nurses must learn to filter quality information for their own learning. In addition, nurses play an important role in teaching clients to safely use health-related information resources.

Ensuring quality of health care information on the Internet is of concern to the government as well as professional groups and organizations. Three approaches have been used to deal with this problem. The first approach is to provide Internet sites with quality health care information. Two examples of government sites that use this approach are *http://www.healthfinder.gov* and *http://www.4women.gov.* A second approach is to develop criteria for identifying quality sites and then label Internet sites that meet these criteria. An example of this approach is *The Health on the Net Foundation Code of Conduct* (HONcode) located at *http://www.hon.ch/.* The third approach is to educate consumers and/or professionals on how to determine the quality of the information that is found. The healthfinder site includes a directory titled *Smart choices: Online health information, evaluating online information* with a number of resources for educating consumers as well as health care professionals. Another example of a group using education is the *Internet Healthcare Coalition*, "the Internet Healthcare Coalition will strive for the following: Well-informed Internet healthcare consumers, professionals, educators, marketers, and both healthcare and mainstream media, as well as public policymakers with regard to the full range of uses of the Internet—current and potential—to deliver high-quality healthcare information and services." (Internet Healthcare Coalition, 1998)

Resources for Teaching Students to Appropriately Use Information.

Appropriate use of information includes synthesizing information from several sources and appropriately identifying resources. For example, an undergraduate nursing student may write a term paper about breast cancer including a section on potential patient reactions to this diagnosis. The information could come from research articles, patient's comments on a list-server, a newspaper article, notes from a nursing class, and even an interview with a patient. Younger students such as freshmen or sophomores often report the information found in each of these resources. Nursing faculty then teach students how to synthesize this information. For example, students can compare the antidotal information with the research information. They can explain how well a newspaper article informed or misinformed consumers. In short, undergraduate students are learning to use critical thinking skills in managing nursing information.

In addition, the student should appropriately footnote the sources of information. Most undergraduate students have a basic understanding of plagiarism, but they are often confused about specific format styles or how to footnote information from multiple sources. Table 3.6 includes several resources that can be used to help students learn proper styles for footnoting Internet resources.

Assessing Learning Outcomes

Measuring student learning includes assessment of student knowledge before the learning experience and measuring achievement of learning after completion of the learning experience. Today students

TABLE 3.6 Web Resources Useful in Teaching Citation of Information Resources

URL	Title and Author
http://www.library.wisc.edu/libraries/Memorial/citing.htm	Internet citation guides compiled by Susan Barribeau, reorganized and updated by Jessica Baumgart
http://www.columbia.edu/cu/cup/cgos/idx_basic.html	Basic CGOS style by Janice R. Walker and Todd Taylor
http://www.library.mcgill.ca/refshelf/citguide.htm	Citation style guides maintained by M. Fransiszyn
http://lcweb2.loc.gov/ammem/ndlpedu/cite.html	Citing electronic sources maintained by Library of Congress
http://funnelweb.utcc.utk.edu/~hoemann/whats.html	Electronic style—What's here developed by George H. Hoemann

enter their collegiate educational experience with a wide range of knowledge and skills related to computer and information literacy. High schools vary greatly in the quality and quantity of computer and information literacy education provided. In addition, many students are older and have graduated from high school years ago. Requiring students to repeat course work that has already been mastered presents problems for both the faculty and the students. It is difficult for the faculty to provide interesting and challenging learning for all students, when some students are just being introduced to the content while other students are ready to move beyond the course content. Students may be either overwhelmed or bored depending on their initial knowledge and skills.

There are several approaches that can be used to assess the previous knowledge and skills of students. A review of a student's transcript or prior course work can provide some insight. However, computer literacy skills previously learned and not reinforced are quickly forgotten. In addition many students who have an excellent knowledge base may have gained their knowledge through other means than traditional credit courses.

An assessment exam or questionnaire can be used to assess the student's current knowledge and/or skill level. These usually take two different approaches. First, students may self-report their level of knowledge. With this approach students review a list of skills (i.e., word processing) and rate their knowledge on a Likert scale from novice to expert (Nelson & Anton, 1995). The problem with this approach is that students may not accurately measure their own knowledge. It is difficult to know what you do not know. A second approach is to use an achievement test. An example of this approach is Tek.Xam, a technology certification exam, developed by the Virginia Foundation for Independent Colleges (VFIC) *http://www.virginiacolleges.org/exam/frame.html.*

An example of an institution using this approach can be seen at the College of Eastern Utah. Information about what is included on the computer literacy exam and how this exam is used can be found at *http://ac.ceu.edu/clexam/.*

NURSING INFORMATICS

Nurses roles include proving client care, planning and implementing educational programs, conducting research, and providing administrative support. Each of these nursing roles requires that nurses effectively manage nursing data, information, knowledge, and wisdom. Nursing informatics is concerned with the use of technology as a tool to manage nursing data, information, knowledge, and wisdom. Technology is now infused into all aspects of health care. This means that all nurses must be prepared to understand and use technology to provide nursing services. However, there is strong documentation that the majority of nurses currently graduating from quality nursing programs across the United States receive little or limited preparation in this vital area.

A recent report issued by National Nursing Informatics Work Group under the direction of The National Advisory Council on Nursing Education and Practice supports this. To define the state of nursing informatics in education and practice, the Work Group completed an extensive review of the literature reported from 1990 to 1997. Fewer than 300 articles were published and only 38 of these reported research findings. From this review the Work Group concluded that, "First, the nursing culture needs to be changed to promote acceptance and use of computer technologies as basic tools for information management and exchange by nurses." They went on to further conclude that "practicing nurses are not necessarily computer competent" and that "more nursing informatics courses are needed" (National Advisory Council on Nursing Education and Practice, 1997). The executive summary from this report can be located at *http://www.hrsa.dhhs.gov/bhpr/DN/nirepex.htm.*

Faculty designing nursing education programs should carefully plan the curriculum including developing a philosophy, program goals, specific courses, as well as rationale and objectives for each course. The courses are carefully organized so that each student moves through a logical program of studies. The specific content and learning experiences are developed so that each student can achieve course goals and, in turn, program goals. There is strong documentation that all programs of nursing need to include nursing informatics content within the educational program. This includes both theoretical content and hands-on experience. The specific approach used will depend on the overall framework and organization of the specific curriculum.

One of the first questions is, should nursing informatics content be integrated into nursing courses or be a separate course? If it is integrated, what approach is used to be sure all students receive the necessary content? If it is a separate course, what approach is used to be sure that students are able to apply concepts from nursing informatics within their nursing courses? Nursing informatics deals with the management of nursing data, information, knowledge, and wisdom. It does not exist as a separate field of study from nursing. Early in their education program, all nursing students begin to work with nursing data. For example, beginning courses usually include an overview of the nursing process with a focus on assessment. This is the point when they should begin to understand different data formats. Students are introduced to nursing diagnosis and the process for developing a nursing diagnosis. As students are being introduced to nursing diagnosis and the correct format for stating these, they are also being introduced to standard languages in nursing. The development and use of standard languages is an important concept for understanding nursing informatics content.

If the faculty decide to include nursing informatics as a separate course, a second question arises. Should nursing informatics be offered as a nursing course or should nursing informatics content be included in an interdisciplinary course? Nursing informatics is one of the discipline-specific areas of informatics under the umbrella of health care informatics. Other examples of discipline-specific informatics areas include medical, dental, and veterinarian informatics. Other very closely related disciplines include health information management and health information technology. Since nursing informatics is part of the interdisciplinary field of health care informatics and can be closely related to health information management, nursing faculty need to consider if they want to use an interdisciplinary approach in designing this aspect of the curriculum. The advantage is that nursing students can understand the role of nursing informatics within the bigger picture. They can gain experience working with health care students and understanding the role of the various health care disciplines in designing and using health care information systems. The disadvantage is that an interdisciplinary approach may include too little content on nursing informatics. This disadvantage can be managed if learning outcomes are well developed and nursing informatics concepts are also integrated into the nursing curriculum.

The third question in planning the appropriate placement of nursing informatics deals with the overlap of computer literacy, information literacy and nursing informatics content. For example, students may have learned how to evaluate information from the Internet, but may not have been introduced to the evaluation of health-related information.

Resources for Teaching Nursing Informatics

There are a number of excellent resources that can be used by faculty teaching students at all levels to develop course rationale, learning objectives, content outlines, clinical and classroom learning experiences, and measures of learning outcomes. The resources presented here focus on the curriculum building process for undergraduate nursing education.

Review of the Literature

Faculty planning for nursing informatics in the curriculum will find a traditional review of the literature very helpful. The resource reference list at the end of this chapter was developed by conducting a series of literature searches on MEDLINE (1991–November, 1999) and CINAHL (1982–June, 1999). These two literature databases are indexed using different subject terms therefore the search was conducted by first identifying the subject terms related to the key words *computers* OR *information systems* OR *informatics.* Second, the key words *undergraduate* OR *baccalaureate* were used to identify the related subject terms. The Boolean AND was then used to combine the articles related to *computer* OR *information system* OR *informatics* with the articles related to *undergraduate* OR *baccalaureate.* The MEDLINE search was limited to nursing. The final result of this search approach included articles dealing with using technology to teach undergraduate nursing students, as well as articles focused on teaching about computers, information systems, and health care informatics. To develop the list presented here, the results of the searches were reviewed. Duplicate results as well as articles about using technology to teach were eliminated.

Resources on the Internet

There are numerous web sites, list-servers, and newsgroups that can be used when teaching nursing informatics content.

Web-pages.

AMIA is a professional organization for health care informatics. It includes several working groups in addition to Nursing Informatics. The American Medical Informatics Association (AMIA) Nursing Informatics Working Group is located at *http://amia-niwg.org/*. The Nursing Informatics Working Group homepage links to two resources that are especially useful in planning curriculum. One link leads to nursing informatics job descriptions with qualifications. Reviewing these can be helpful in developing course and/or program learning outcomes. In addition, this site includes a link to several nursing informatics programs and/or courses. These sites provide examples of curriculum plans as well as syllabi for individual courses. Table 3.7 includes several examples of undergraduate course syllabi that can be located on the Internet.

List-servers.

There are at least two list-servers that are especially useful to faculty planning for nursing informatics in the undergraduate curriculum. The first of these is Nrsinged. The subscription address for this list server is *listserv@ulkyvm.louisville.edu*. Most discussions on this list focus on nursing education in total. These participants are interested in technology and its impact on nursing education. They can be an excellent resource when making curriculum decisions.

The second list server is nrsing-l. This list focuses on nursing informatics in practice and education. The discussions often deal with many of the practical and theorical issues experienced by nurses working in the field of nursing informatics. Postings to this list are archived back to May 1991. The URL for subscribing to the list and for searching the archives is *http://mailman.amia.org/listinfo/nrsing-l.*

Publications from Professional Organizations.

The American Nurses Association identified nursing informatics as a nursing specialty in 1992. As part of this process they defined the scope and standards of practice. References outlining the scope and standards of practice are especially useful in planning for nursing informatics in the undergraduate curriculum.

TABLE 3.7 Examples of Undergraduate Syllabi from the Web.

URL	Course title and name of faculty on syllabus
http://www.uvm.edu/~nursing/prnu112.html	Introduction to nursing informatics developed by Jack Yensen
http://vms.cc.wmich.edu/~young/outline.htm	Information systems for health care professionals developed by Kathy Young, M.A., R.N.C.
http://www.indwes.edu/Academics/Nursing/s224.htm	NUR224 NURSING INFORMATICS developed by Barbara A. Ihrke, R.N., M.S.
http://nursing.rutgers.edu/nursing/syllabi/nursing_informatics.html	Nursing informatics developed by Rachel Wilson, M.S., R.N., C.S., F.N.P.
http://www.athabascau.ca/html/syllabi/nurs/nurs491.htm	NURS 491: Nursing informatics no faculty identified on the syllabus
http://www.rockhurst.edu/academic_programs/nursing/infomat3.html	Nursing informatics syllabus developed by Martha Bogart, R.N., M.S.N., Karen Cooper, R.N., M.S.N., and Sheryl Max, R.N., M.N.

The Scope of Practice for Nursing Informatics by the American Nurses Association (ANA, 1994) defines the scope of practice. It outlines the relationship between nursing informatics and nursing as well as other informatics disciplines. Key to the development of undergraduate nursing programs is the fact that the document identifies four competencies required for graduates of basic nursing programs. These include:

1. Identify, collect, and record data relevant to the nursing care of patients;
2. Analyze and interpret patient and nursing information as part of the planning for and provision of nursing services;
3. Employ health care informatics applications designed for the clinical practice of nursing;

4. Implement public and institutional policies related to privacy, confidentiality, and security of information.

Each of these competencies indicate nursing informatics content that should be included in undergraduate nursing curriculum. For example, in order to achieve number 3 above, students need experience using health care information systems in clinical settings. To achieve number 4, undergraduate students need experience using passwords and understanding how passwords are used to secure confidential on-line data.

The preparation for an informatics nurse is a bachelor's degree and additional knowledge and experience in the field of informatics. This document lists 12 requisite competencies and six additional skills. Each of these competencies builds on knowledge that is gained in an undergraduate program and therefore has implications for content in the undergraduate curriculum. For example, one of the competencies is testing and evaluating applications for nursing. Prerequisite knowledge for this competency includes understanding how nurses work with nursing information, critical thinking skills, and experience using health-care applications in providing care.

Standards of Practice for Nursing Informatics by the American Nurses Association (ANA, 1995) identifies the practice standards, the professional performance standards, and the domain standards for a nurse engaged in nursing informatics practice. These standards apply to a nurse who has a baccalaureate degree in nursing along with additional education and experience in nursing informatics. The graduate of a baccalaureate program would not be expected to meet these standards without the additional education. However since that education is continuing education and not a master's degree, a graduate of a baccalaureate program is expected to have the background necessary to benefit from that continuing education. For example, the student should be able to read and understand the standards. This means that he/she would need to be familiar with the terminology and concepts included in this document.

The Scope of Practice for Nursing Informatics and *The Standards of Practice for Nursing Informatics* developed by the ANA provide the conceptual framework for the nursing informatics certification exam offered by the American Nurses Credentialing Center. Information about the exam including the eight content areas can be found at *http://www.ana.org/ancc/index.htm.*

National Reports

Because health care and technology are changing at such a rapid rate national reports can become outdated quickly. However some of these national reports do include conceptual frameworks and planning directions that are important to faculty building an undergraduate curriculum.

Bringing Health Care Online (U.S Congress, Office of Technical Assessment, 1995) This government report "identifies key technologies and shows how they are being used to communicate clinical information, simplify administration of health care delivery, assess the quality of health care, inform the decision making of providers and administrators, and support the delivery of health care at a distance" (page iii). This report can be used to identify clinical experiences and theory content for the undergraduate curriculum. For example, page 13 includes a figure with information about applications in telecommunication that have been adapted or planned in the near future. Ask-a-nurse referral service is ranked 5th, yet few undergraduate curriculums include information or student experiences providing health education using telecommunication.

A National Informatics Agenda for Nursing Education and Practice (National Advisory Council on Nursing Education and Practice, 1997) was referred to in the introduction to this section of the chapter. The first recommendation in this report reads as follows:
Educate nursing students and practicing nurses in core informatics content. Federal resources should promote the inclusion of core informatics skills and knowledge leading to competency in nursing undergraduate, graduate, and continuing education programs.
The recommendation provides strong rationale for a curriculum revision that includes informatics content within the nursing curriculum. In addition, the report includes five informatics education models with the names of universities and schools that have implemented these models. Models 2, 3, and 4 are directly applicable to undergraduate programs. Initial identification of core computing skills and informatics content is provided in section IV of the report. However, the report does not provide a complete description of all core content. Additional resources are needed by the faculty.

If nurses are to direct the flow of nursing data, information, knowledge, and wisdom, they must understand factors that influence this flow. *Next-Generation Nursing Information Systems* (Zielstorff, Hudgings,

Grove, & The National Commission on Nursing Implementation Project, 1993) represents the work of over 200 individuals, groups, and organizations. The report includes rationale for including nursing informatics content in the undergraduate curriculum as well as essential content. For example, students need to know and be able to use standard languages and minimum databases that are used in patient care. This reference includes several figures that can be used in teaching the levels and types of nursing data as well as the interrelationships between nursing data, information, and knowledge.

SUGGESTED NURSING INFORMATICS CONTENT FOR UNDERGRADUATE STUDENTS

The following is offered as a starting point for faculty who are developing course objectives and learning experiences.

Potential Objectives

1. Recognize historical perspectives of computer applications in health care.
2. Analyze the role of the nursing informatics specialist including scope and standards of practice.
3. Discuss model and theories used in managing nursing data, information, and knowledge.
4. Apply database concepts and principles to the management of health care data, information, knowledge, and wisdom
5. Describe various ways that automation can support nursing administration, patient/client care, education, and research.
6. Explain the life cycle of a health care information system including the role of nurses in each step of the cycle.
7. Describe various health care information management roles and positions including their relationship to nursing.
8. Use concepts from telecommunication, networking, and integration to describe integrated health care information systems.
9. Analyze the role of technical, professional, and clinical standards impacting nursing information systems including the use of standard nursing languages and minimum databases.
10. Apply ethical and legal principles in using automated health care information systems to provide patient care.

Potential Course Content

1. Introduction:
   A. Evolution of the nursing informatics specialty
   B. Early educational, clinical, administrative systems used in nursing
   C. Initial educational programs
   D. The role of professional organizations
2. Theories and models for nursing information systems
   A. Models for nursing information systems
   B. Theories supporting nursing information systems
   C. Nursing theories and information systems
   D. Dictionary, thesaurus, classification, and nomenclature
3. Nursing information resources
   A. Locating information
   B. Information and knowledge structures
   C. Evaluation of information
   D. Evaluation tools
4. Database management concepts in health care
   A. Database models
   B. Data warehouses
   C. Decision support systems
5. Information systems used in health care
   A. Hospital information systems
   B. Departmental information systems
   C. Specialty information systems (i.e., OR systems.)
   D. Integrated delivery systems
6. Life cycle of a health care information system
   A. Assessment and identification of needs
   B. System selection
   C. Systems implementation
   D. Evaluating and upgrading health care information systems
7. Nursing information systems supporting patient care
   A. Functions of clinical information systems
   B. Automation and the nursing process
   C. Interrelationship of nursing information systems with other clinical systems
8. Administrative systems used in nursing
   A. Clinical, personal, inventory and financial data in nursing
   B. Using information systems in administrative decision making

9. Information systems used in patient/client education
   A. Designing educational materials
   B. Using technology to present health care information
   C. Consumer informatics and the Internet
10. Information systems in nursing research
    A. Research questions in nursing informatics
    B. Using technology to support nursing research
11. Data integrity, security and confidentiality
    A. Integrity, security, privacy and confidentiality
    B. Impact of automated systems on privacy and confidentiality
12. Security and Disaster Planning
    A. Prevention: Information and system security
    B. Disaster plan and recovery
13. Accreditation, regulations, and standards
    A. Professional standards including language
    B. Accreditation standards
    C. Technical standards
    D. Federal regulations
14. Computer-based patient records
    A. CPR recommendations
    B. CPRI
15. Issues, trends, and future directions
    A. Strategic planning process
    B. New technology (voice recognition.)
    C. Patient access to on-line medical records

FACULTY PREPARATION

Both the National League for Nursing Accrediting Commission (NLNAC) and the Commission on Collegiate Nursing Education (CCNE) include in their accrediting standards, a statement related to faculty qualifications. For example, the NLNAC includes the following:

The program has qualified and credentialed faculty appropriate to accomplish its purposes and strengthen its educational effectiveness. (NLNAC, 1999)

From both of these professional groups one can conclude that the faculty planning and implementing nursing informatics content in the undergraduate curriculum should be qualified in nursing informatics. The type of qualifications needed in nursing informatics do not differ from the qualifications within any of the other nursing specialties. That is, the faculty should have additional academic preparation related to nursing informatics beyond that provided in their undergraduate program. There are several other chapters in this book dealing with continuing and graduate education in nursing informatics. These chapters provide a basis for identifying the educational and practical experiences of qualified faculty.

SUMMARY

This chapter has focused on assessing, planning, implementing, and evaluating nursing informatics content in the undergraduate nursing curriculum. The interrelationships between computer literacy, information literacy, and nursing informatics were presented.

Resources for developing course rationale, descriptions, objectives, learning experiences and measuring outcomes were reviewed. Suggested course objectives and content were outlined. The need for qualified faculty was stressed.

REFERENCES

American Nurses Association (1995). *Standards of practice for nursing informatics.* Washington, D.C.: American Nurses Publishing.

American Nurses Association's Task Force on the Scope of Practice for Nursing Informatics (1994). *The scope of practice for nursing informatics.* Washington, D. C: American Nurses Publishing.

Computer Literacy, *Microsoft(r) Encarta(r) 97 Encyclopedia.* 1993–1996 Microsoft Corporation.

Internet Healthcare Coalition (1998). *Mission statement.* Retrieved September 16, 1999. [On-line] Available: *http://www.ihc.net/about/mission.html.*

Joos, I., Whitman, N., Smith, M., & Nelson R, (2000). *Computers in small bytes: A workbook for healthcare professionals* (3rd ed.). Sudbury, Massachusetts: Jones and Bartlett Publishers.

National Advisory Council on Nursing Education and Practice (1997). *A national informatics agenda for nursing education and practice.* Washington, D.C.: Bureau of Health Professions, U.S. Department of Health and Human Services.

The National Commission on Excellence in Education (1983). *A Nation at risk: The imperative for educational reform a report to the nation and the Secretary of Education United States Department of Education.* Retrieved September 10, 1999. [On-line] available: *http://www.ed. gov/pubs/NatAtRisk/title.html.*

The National League for Nursing Accrediting Commission (1999). *1999 Accreditation Manual.* Retrieved October 5, 1999. [On-line] available: *http://www.accrediting-comm-nlnac.org/.*

Nelson, R. & Anton, B. (1996). A format for surveying computer related learning needs in health care settings. Computers in Nursing. May/June 14(3), 150–151.

Ronald, J. S., & Skiba, D. (1987). *Guidelines for basic computer education in nursing.* New York: National League for Nursing.

Saba, V., & McCormick, K. A. (1995). *Essentials of Computers for Nurses* (2nd ed.), p. 29. New York: McGraw Hill

Technology Competency of Graduates in *Virginia Commonwealth University's Restructuring Report for 1997–98.* Retrieved September 21, 1999. [On-line] available: *http://www.vcu.edu/provost/restructuring978/technologycompetency.html.*

U.S Congress, Office of Technical Assessment, (1995). *Bringing health care online: The role of information technologies.* OTA-ITC-624 Washington, D.C.: U. S. Government Printing Office. September.

Zielstorff, R., Hudgings, C. I., Grove, S., & The National Commission on Nursing Implementation Project (1993). *Next-Generation nursing information systems: Essential characteristics for professional practice.* Washington D.C.: American Nursing Publishing.

A RESOURCE REFERENCE LIST

Arnold, J. M. (1996). Nursing informatics educational needs. *Computers in Nursing, 14*(6), 333–9, Nov–Dec.

Bachman, J. A., & Panzarine, S. (1998). Enabling student nurses to use the information superhighway. *Journal of Nursing Education, 37*(4), 155–61, Apr.

Barnett, D. E. (1995). Informing the nursing professions about IT. *Medinfo, 8 Pt, 2,* 1316–20.

Bird, D., & Roberts, P. M. (1998). The role of library and information services in the modular curriculum. *Nurse Education Today, 18*(7), 583–91Oct.

Carter, B. E., & Axford, R. L. (1993). Assessment of computer learning needs and priorities of registered nurses practicing in hospitals. *Computers in Nursing, 11*(3), 122–6, May–Jun.

Carty, B., & Rosenfeld, P. (1998). From computer technology to information technology. Findings from a national study of nursing education. *Computers in Nursing, 16*(5), 259–65, Sep–Oct.

Cheek, J., Gillham, D., & Mills, P. (1998). Using clinical databases in tertiary nurse education: An innovative approach of computer technology. *Nurse Education Today, 18*(2), 153–7, Feb.

Curl, L., Hoehn, J., & Theile, J. R. (1988). Computer applications in nursing: A new course in the curriculum. *Computers in Nursing, 6*(6), 263–8, Nov–Dec.

Curry, P., Elliott, D., Wheeler, E., & Guhde, R. (1992). Implementing an automated care planning system in a nursing curriculum. In *Computer applications in nursing education and practice* (Arnold, J. M., et al.). National League for Nursing Publications. NLN PUBL ** 1992 #14–2406 (pp. 133–7).

Curtis, K. L. (1996). Teaching roles of librarians in nursing education. *Bulletin of the Medical Library Association, 84*(3), 416–22, Jul.

Davis, G. C. (1987). Keeping the focus on nursing. *Nursing Outlook, 35*(6), 285–7, Nov–Dec.

Edwardson, S. R., & Pejsa, J. (1993). A computer assisted tutorial for applications of computer spreadsheets in nursing financial management. *Computers in Nursing, 11*(4), 169–75, 1993, Jul–Aug.

Fox, L. M., Richter, J. M., & White, N. (1989). Pathways to information literacy. *Journal of Nursing Education, 28*(9), 422–5, Nov.

Fox, L. M., Richter, J. M., & White, N. E. (1996). A multidimensional evaluation of a nursing information-literacy program. *Bulletin of the Medical Library Association, 84*(2), 182–90, Apr.

Francis, B. W., & Fisher, C. C. (1995). Multilevel library instruction for emerging nursing roles. *Bulletin of the Medical Library Association, 83*(4), 492–8, Oct.

Glancey, T. S., Vessey, J. A., & Rhodes, G. (1992). Computer graphics and developmental theory: A powerful partnership. *Computers in Nursing, 10*(2), 81–4, Mar–Apr.

Goodman, J., & Blake, J. (1996). Multimedia courseware. Transforming the classroom. *Computers in Nursing, 14*(5), 287–96; quiz 297–8, Sep–Oct.

Graveley, E., & Fullerton, J. T. (1998). Incorporating electronic-based and computer-based strategies: Graduate nursing courses in administration. *Journal of Nursing Education, 37*(4), 186–8, Apr.

Graves, J. R., Amos, L. K., Huether, S., Lange, L. L., & Thompson, C. B. (1995). Description of a graduate program in clinical nursing informatics. *Computers in Nursing, 13*(2), 60–70, Mar–Apr.

Hall, E. (1995). Highlighting emerging roles and enduring values: Information management in nursing education. *Bulletin of the Medical Library Association, 83*(4), 490–1, Oct.

Hasman, A. (1994). Education and training in health informatics. *Computer Methods & Programs in Biomedicine, 45*(1–2), 41–3, Oct.

Heller, B. R., Romano, C. A., Damrosch, S., & Parks, P. (1985). Computer applications in nursing: implications for the curriculum. *Computers in Nursing, 3*(1), 14–22, Jan–Feb.

Hilgenberg, C., & Damery, L. (1994). Introduction to an automated hospital information system in baccalaureate education: a pilot project. *Journal of Nursing Education, 33*(8), 378–80, Oct.

Hinegardner, P. G., & Lansing, P. S. (1994). Nursing informatics programs at the University of Maryland at Baltimore. *Bulletin of the Medical Library Association, 82*(4), 441–3, Oct.

Hovenga, E. J. (1998). Health and medical informatics education for nurses and health service managers. *International Journal of Medical Informatics, 50*(1–3), 21–9, Jun.

Johnson, J. Y. J. (1995). Curricular trends in accredited generic baccalaureate nursing programs across the United States. *Journal of Nursing Education, 34*(2), 53–60, Feb.

Kilmon, C. A. (1995). Computerized approaches to teaching nurse practitioner students. *Pediatric Nursing, 22*(1), 16–8, Jan–Feb.

Kooker, B. M., & Richardson, S. S. (1994). Information revolution in nursing and health care: Educating for tomorrow's challenge. *Seminars for Nurse Managers, 2*(2), 79–84, Jun.

Lawless, K. A. (1993). Nursing informatics as a needed emphasis in graduate nursing administration education: The student perspective. *Computers in Nursing, 11*(6), 263–8, Nov–Dec.

Lewis, D., Watson, J. E., & Newfield, S. (1997). Implementing instructional technology. Strategies for success. *Computers in Nursing, 15*(4), 187–90, Jul–Aug.

Mantas, J. (1998). Developing curriculum in nursing informatics in Europe. *International Journal of Medical Informatics, 50*(1–3), 123–32, Jun.

Marin, H. F. (1998). Nursing Informatics in Brazil. A Brazilian experience. *Computers in Nursing, 16*(6), 327–32, Nov–Dec.

Mastrian, K. G., & McGonigle, D. (1999). Using technology-based assignments to promote critical thinking. *Nurse Educator, 24*(1), 45–7, Jan–Feb.

Noll, M. L., & Murphy, M. A. (1993). Integrating nursing informatics into a graduate research course. *Journal of Nursing Education, 32*(7), 332–4, Sep.

Poirrier, G. P., Wills, E. M., Broussard, P. C., & Payne, R. L. (1996). Nursing information systems: applications in nursing curricula. *Nurse Educator, 21*(1), 18–22, Jan–Feb.

Pollack, C. D., & Diers, D. (1996). Data as textbook. *Computers in Nursing, 14*(1), 31–6; quiz 37–8, Jan–Feb.

Saranto, K., & Leino-Kilpi, H. (1997). Computer literacy in nursing: Developing the information technology syllabus in nursing education. *Journal of Advanced Nursing, 25*(2), 377–85, Feb.

Saranto, K., & Tallberg, M. (1998). Nursing informatics in nursing education: A challenge to nurse teachers. *Nurse Education Today, 18*(1), 79–87, Jan.

Saver, C. (1994). Nursing informatics education. *Nursing Spectrum, 4*(19), 9, Sep 19. D.C./Baltimore Metro Edition.

Skiba, D. J. (1997). Nursing education to celebrate learning. *N & HC Perspectives on Community, 18*(3), 124–9, 148, May–Jun.

Stamler, L. L., Thomas, B., & McMahon, S. (1999). Nursing students respond to a computer assignment. *Journal of Professional Nursing, 15*(1), 52–8, Jan–Feb.

Summers, S. (1992). High technology impact on nursing education. *Kansas Nurse, 67*(12), 5–6, Nov–Dec.

Thiele, J. E. (1988). There's a computer in the curriculum! *Computers in Nursing,* 6(1), 37–40, Jan–Feb.

Travis, L., & Brennan, P. F. (1998). Information science for the future: An innovative nursing informatics curriculum. *Journal of Nursing Education,* 37(4), 162–8, Apr.

Travis, L. L., Hoehn, B., Spees, C., Hribar, K., & Youngblut, J. (1992). Supporting collaboration through a nursing informatics curriculum stage II. *Proceedings—The Annual Symposium on Computer Applications in Medical Care,* 419–23.

Travis, L. L., Hudak, C. A., & Brennan, P. F. (1995). Summative evaluation of a baccalaureate nursing informatics curriculum. *Annual Symposium on Computer Applications in Medical Care,* 484–7.

Travis, L. L., & Youngblut, J. (1993). Supporting patient centered computing through an undergraduate nursing informatics curriculum stage III. *Proceedings—The Annual Symposium on Computer Applications in Medical Care,* 757–61.

Travis, L. L., Youngblut, J., & Brennan, P. F. (1994). The effects of an undergraduate nursing informatics curriculum on students' knowledge and attitudes. *Proceedings—The Annual Symposium on Computer Applications in Medical Care,* 41–5.

Turner, S. L., & Bentley, G. W. (1998). A meaningful health assessment course for baccalaureate nursing students. *Nursing Connections,* 11(2), 5–12, Summer.

Vanderbeek, J., & Beery, T. A. (1998). A blueprint for an undergraduate healthcare informatics course. *Nurse Educator,* 23(1), 15–9, Jan–Feb.

Vanderbeek, J., Ulrich, D., Jaworski, R., Werner, L., Hergert, D., Beery, T., & Baas, L. (1994). Bringing nursing informatics into the undergraduate classroom. *Computers in ursing,* 12(5), 227–31, Sep–Oct.

Williams, R. D., & Benedict, S. (1990). RN education flexibility utilizing laptop computers. *Computers in Nursing,* 8(5), 201–3, Sep–Oct.

Wood, C. L. (1992). A computer-based AIDS education program for nursing students. *Computers in Nursing,* 10(1), 25–35, Jan–Feb.

Wood, D. (1998). Effects of educational focus on a graduate nurse's initial choice of practice area. *Journal of Professional Nursing,* 14(4), 214–9, Jul–Aug.

4

Nursing Informatics: Graduate Education

Barbara Carty

Health care informatics, a relatively new and expanding area of study, continues to grow as a result of the ubiquitous presence of information and communication technology in all aspects of the health care delivery system. Rapidly evolving ways in which healthcare information is acquired, stored, retrieved, and used is dramatically altering the context of healthcare encounters and the structure of the healthcare industry. The emphasis on data driven decisions within a managed care environment is determining to a great extent how care is allocated, evaluated, and financed. All of these factors are propelling the rapid evolution of health informatics.

Nursing is in a pivotal position to provide practitioners who will work in the interdisciplinary field of health informatics. Crucial to the contribution of nursing is the responsibility to articulate the domain of nursing within this interdisciplinary arena. Nursing informatics specialists on a graduate level will influence the design and development of clinical systems, promote the integration of nursing knowledge in systems, and apply research methods in the process, storage, and retrieval of nursing and patient care data within an interdisciplinary environment.

Although nursing informatics is a relatively new specialty, the need for nurses with knowledge in the area of informatics will increase rapidly as the demand for health professionals with expertise in health care systems far exceeds the supply in the next decade. In a recent survey, the Department of Labor identified the most rapidly growing areas for future employment. Of the top ten areas, six were in information services and four were in health-related fields (Dept. of Labor, 1999).

This chapter will explore three major dynamics operating in the area of nursing informatics today: 1) the current status of graduate nursing informatics education, 2) the domain of nursing informatics education within an interdisciplinary framework, and 3) the description of graduate informatics content as illustrated by a specific program.

CURRENT STATUS OF NURSING INFORMATICS EDUCATION FOR THE INFORMATICS NURSE

In 1994, the American Nurses Association developed the scope of practice for nursing informatics and in 1995 established standards for practice. Since the inception of its first credentialing exam in 1995, 275 nurses have been credentialed in the specialty of nursing informatics (ANCC, 1999). Although a new specialty, this number underscores the lack of nurses prepared in the specialty. The current credentialing criteria do not require a master's degree but nurses must have a minimum of 2,000 hours of practice in the field or have completed 12 hours of course work with 1,000 hours of practice within 5 years of taking the credentialing exam. The informatics nurse specialist (INS), prepared on the master's level, has been recognized as the acceptable level of preparation. Leaders in the field and the profession have endorsed this position (ANA, 1995; Gassert, 1998; National Advisory Council on Nurse Education and Practice, 1997).

Compounding the need for nurses with advanced specialized skills and knowledge in the area of informatics is the paucity of education programs to prepare nurses in the specialty. A nationwide study of nursing programs in the country indicated that less than one-third of the schools addressed nursing informatics in the curriculum and only 19 (9%) schools indicated that nursing informatics was offered as a separate course (Carty & Rosenfeld, 1998). A recent visit to the American Medical Informatics Association (AMIA) Nursing Informatics Workgroup website (*http://amia-niwg.org*) which provides a listing of education programs in nursing informatics reports a similar scarcity of programs: five schools with a specialty in nursing informatics, seven schools with graduate or undergraduate courses, and eight schools with a concentration/minor in nursing informatics.

The variety of curricula and methodological approaches among these programs underscores the unique and unusual composition of the specialty. Some programs have an interdisciplinary focus, offering courses with other departments, including computer science, management, and medical informatics. Some have a strong nursing emphasis supplementing faculty with specialists from other areas such as medical informatics, clinical informaticists, and management systems engineers. The emphasis on clinical experience also differs with a range of hours from 60 to 600 and with variable requirements for clinical projects (Spring AMIA, 1999).

AN EMERGING SPECIALTY

The diversity and innovation of the approaches to graduate nursing informatics education underscores the evolving nature of a discipline, which is intricately integrated with a rapidly evolving technology and information infrastructure. The revolution in connectivity, technology, and communication is transforming the way we interact as a national and global society (Kelly, 1999). Subsequent technological effects are altering health care delivery and transactions among the providers and recipients of the system.

Why, then, are there so few programs and educational opportunities when there is and will continue to be a growing demand for nurses in this specialty? Faculty development has been cited as a major factor in the ability of schools to offer and prepare nurses in the specialty (AMIA Nursing Working Group Meeting, 1999; Arnold, 1996; Carty & Rosenfeld, 1998). The lack of prepared faculty for informatics programs can be attributed to limited funding to educate nurses and to support programs of research in the area. The recent provision by the Division of Nursing to support informatics education on the graduate level is a much needed reform. Up until now, the majority of nurses practicing in the field have been self-directed, taking courses in a number of disciplines in addition to benefiting from on-the-job training (Arnold, 1996; Carty, 1994).

The lack of explicit competencies for nurse informatics specialists is another major drawback in the recognition of the specialty. Current efforts are being made to address this need (see Gassert & Staggers, chapter 3). A phenomena not often encountered in other specialties is the rapid advancement and acceleration of technology. Knowledge of systems can often become obsolete in a very short time and great expenses are incurred in the purchase and maintenance of computer-based technology. In fact, infrastructure and personnel resources have been identified as essential factors in implementing informatics content (Carty & Phillip, in press). The expertise needed to develop and implement nursing informatics courses and programs is often compounded by an inability to separate the technology and hardware issues from the theory and information content of informatics. It is not unusual for schools, departments, and nursing programs to expect the informatics specialist role to be one of implementing a computer learning lab or distance education program. The use of technology to deliver informatics or other curricula content is the domain of educational technology and also raises issues of faculty development and competencies. It is not, however, the domain of informatics. The ability to discern the difference between technology as a tool and information as a commodity is essential.

Nursing informatics as a specialty is clearly evolving and becoming more defined as researchers and specialists interpret and elucidate the domain of practice and research, and organizations and credentialing agencies specify the scope, standards, and competencies of practice (AACN, 1998; ANA, 1994, 1995; Gassert & Staggers, in press).

THE DOMAIN OF NURSING INFORMATICS

A definition of nursing informatics has evolved over the past 10 years. Initially, Corcoran and Graves defined nursing informatics as the management and processing of nursing data into nursing information, and nursing data and information into nursing knowledge for the purpose of patient care (Graves and Corcoran Perry, 1989). Subsequent definitions have expanded the concept of nursing informatics to incorporate other disciplines, including computer science, information science, and nursing science. A model by Turley (1996) incorporates cognitive science into the nursing informatics model. The inclusion of cognitive science has been echoed by Ribbons (1998) in nursing informatics and Patel & Kaufman (1998) in medical informatics. As more increasingly complex informatics strategies are developed in education, nursing, and patient care, the science of cognition will inform much of the research. This is particularly relevant to the area of decision support systems and complex learning systems.

As with any new specialty, time is needed to articulate the domain and develop a research body to support the practice. Since the development of the first nursing informatics program (Heller, Romano, Moray, & Gassert, 1989) much progress has been made by specialists who have researched areas as diverse as vocabularies, standards, decision support, and theory (Brennan, 1995; Brennan, Lorenson, & Ruland, 1997; Daly, et al. 1997; Graves, et al., 1995; Goossen, et al., 1998; Henry, et al., 1998; Maas, Johnson & Mooched, 1996; McClosky & Bulechek, 1996; McCormick, 1994; Ozbolt, 1996; Saba, 1992). These intense efforts have produced significant results in 1) the identification of the domain of nursing within the discipline of informatics, 2) the articulation of nursing within a health informatics framework, and 3) the incorporation of informatics into the nursing curricula. It is in the work of defining nursing vocabularies and adopting standards for systems that informatics has made one of its most important contributions to the profession of nursing and the body of knowledge of nursing informatics. The ability of nurses to articulate, record, communicate, and research care processes and patient outcomes is vital to the recognition of the profession. The ability, in turn, to develop and design systems, that capture this same data and information, is essential to the viability of the profession within an information intensive and driven industry. The question is how to best prepare advanced informatics nurses?

Graduate Preparation in Nursing Informatics

Graduate or advanced preparation requires the identification of a specialized body of knowledge. If one acknowledges the "newness" of the area of informatics, then the conundrum of discipline specific and/or interdisciplinary content is understandable. Most new disciplines borrow, or absorb from prior developed bodies of knowledge. Uniquely important in the development of the body of nursing informatics is the influence of technology. Technology as defined within the context of today's society is both ubiquitous and invasive; " it is the matrix of our society" (Kelly, 1999). Therefore in any subsequent discussion of nursing informatics, the influence and integration of technology is assumed and not discussed as a separate entity.

The most prominent endorsement for graduate informatics preparation was supported by the National Advisory Panel on Nurse Education and Practice (1997).

Among the recommendations addressed by the council were:

- Identification of core informatics content
- Preparation of advanced informatics nurses
- Preparation of faculty in informatics
- Collaboration on informatics projects

A PROTOTYPE GRADUATE INFORMATICS PROGRAM

The development and implementation of a specialized, graduate curriculum requires the identification of graduate nursing informatics content and in-depth planning, research, and collaboration. In 1996, the Division of Nursing at New York University committed to the development of a graduate nursing informatics program with a strong emphasis on clinical applications and experience. The plan was to establish a collaborative model of academicians and clinicians in nursing informatics with a strong clinical focus on "real life" clinical projects to augment theory. The theoretical underpinnings for the curriculum expand on the Graves and Corcoran Perry (1989) model of data, information, and knowledge. (See Figure 4.1.)

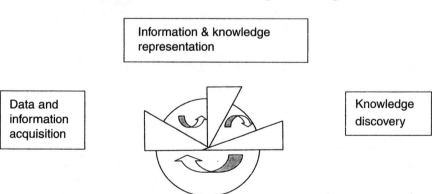

FIGURE 4.1 Nursing informatics model.

The model supported by the New York University informatics program proposes an interpretation of data, information, and knowledge that is complex and nonlinear. It is a direct outgrowth of two important developments: 1) the ability to transform and model knowledge in complex, interactive systems, and 2) the advances that have been made in the researching of nursing language and taxonomies.

The model is recursive, dynamic, and interactive (in press). As supported by the model, the concept of data, information, and knowledge can be introduced in the baccalaureate level of education. The more advanced concepts of information and knowledge representation are supported throughout the graduate courses in the informatics program. The knowledge discovery content is introduced at the graduate level, but is more appropriately addressed in-depth within the domain of the informatics researcher and doctoral study.

To support the model, courses in database design and decision support are introduced and students are required to design a clinical project that involves the development of a decision support system within the context of a clinical situation. The incorporation of nursing language and nursing practice guidelines are requisite to the project. The proposed model is being simultaneously articulated and evaluated in an evolving curriculum.

In addition to identifying a model of informatics, a key to success in the planning for the graduate program was endorsement from both administration and faculty. This presupposed an understanding of the focus of the program, including the emphasis on data, information, knowledge, and clinical informatics applications as opposed to tangential areas such as computer literacy and educational technology. Research indicates that faculty lack a knowledge and understanding of nursing informatics (Arnold, 1996; Carty & Rosenfeld, 1998). Therefore, 2 years prior to the development of the nursing informatics program a strategy that involved faculty development, and the creation of an informatics infrastructure was initiated.

Informatics Infrastructure

First and foremost, an extensive plan for faculty development and education was implemented. This was considered "laying the groundwork" for the informatics program. The plan included the development of a technology-based infrastructure and the initiation of faculty workshops. All faculty were provided with computers, a local area network was established and connected to the large and robust university Intranet, and a network manager was hired. Policies were created for electronic communications and an infrastructure was established that would promote and support an informatics curriculum. The strategic role of the one nursing informatics faculty during this time was that of facilitator and innovator. Rogers (1995) has identified the innovator role as key to the successful transition and change in an environment. The high visibility of this role also legitimized and demonstrated the expertise of the informatics faculty member. In addition to the above strategies, other educational approaches included the development of a graduate core course in nursing informatics and guest appearances in other courses to describe the role of the nurse informaticist. These approaches helped to inform and educate both faculty and students of the domain of nursing informatics. In addition, a continuing education program in nursing informatics was initiated and is offered on an annual basis. This annual event continues to raise the visibility of nursing informatics within the community and the region.

Curriculum Development

One year prior to the development of the program, a panel of national experts in nursing informatics was convened to provide input into the curriculum and course content. Program objectives were developed and a curriculum was designed. The decision was made to develop five (5) nursing informatics courses, including the modification of an introductory course in nursing informatics, which was currently offered as an elective. The other four (4) courses were to have a clinical component of a minimum of 8 hours (1 day per week). The final course, an integration course requires 2 days a week of clinical practicum. All of the nursing informatics concentration courses are offered in the division of nursing. Thorough discussion on the course content resulted in the development of the following courses:

- Nursing Informatics: An Introduction
- Assessment and Analysis of Clinical Information Systems
- Decision Support in Clinical Information Systems

- Implementation, Management, and Evaluation of Clinical Information Systems
- Informatics Integration

As previously stated, the courses support a complex model of data, information and knowledge acquisition, representation, and discovery (see Figure 4.1). The system analysis and assessment course provide the foundation for data and information acquisition. The decision support and system evaluation courses integrate the concepts of information and knowledge representation. The integration course allows the student to explore the construct of knowledge discovery. It lays the foundation for the informatics researcher in the area of knowledge discovery, particularly through data mining techniques. It is through postgraduate and doctoral work that the area of knowledge discovery is further pursued.

Since real life clinical experiences in decision support are at a premium, laboratory exercises with software tools that simulate the development and application of decision support and analysis are required. For these projects, students are required to incorporate practice standards, nursing language, and interventions into a decision support model. Students also work with clinicians to format large clinical data sets to discover patterns, examine outcomes, and determine effectiveness of care. Projects have included modeling longitudinal data sets to determine outcomes of asthma patients across settings, formatting and structuring data sets of clients with decubiti, falls, and pain management. Using real clinical data, students have developed prototype relational databases to assist clinicians to make informed decisions and incorporate best practice methods into care protocols.

The final integration course employs a clinical case study method. We have also incorporated Blackboard, an interactive distance learning platform in this course and different infomatics faculty "visit" the class on a weekly basis. In depth clinical informatics case studies are discussed and examined with the visiting experts. Feedback indicates the students find this format invaluable in understanding real life informatics situation.

In addition to the informatics courses, all students are required to take six core courses and two electives to complete the master degree. For the electives, students may select from the following departments: computer science, public health and policy, business, or interactive technology. Students in the generic master's track take a total of 45 credits, students in the postmaster's track take 21 credits. Prior to admission, all students enrolled in the program are expected to demonstrate a level of basic computer literacy, own a computer, and have at least 1 year clinical experience. As demonstrated by the current student profile, students far exceed these minimal requirements. The average age of the students is 36 years and the mean years of experience is 14.

Clinical Integration

Almost 1 year after the first class was admitted, there are two full-time faculty and three adjunct faculty. Based on the decision to implement an interdisciplinary focus, while maintaining the emphasis on the domain of nursing, the adjunct faculty and guest lecturers represent medical informatics, information technology, and management information systems as well as nursing informatics. The students are exposed to a variety of faculty as well as clinical environments. They are individually mentored for their clinical experience and at any one time they are involved in projects on database design, project development, system implementation, automation of clinical data including vocabularies, coding, decision support, and evaluation and quality assessment of systems. Students are required to complete a total of 600 hours of clinical experience in the program; clinical settings include tertiary, primary, community, and home health care. Key to the success of the clinical experience is the close collaboration between clinical informaticists (preceptors) practicing in the field of informatics, faculty teaching courses, and students. During any semester students are involved with up to seven to eight agencies. As structured within the courses, students report on clinical projects and share clinical experiences and encounters. As a result, all students benefit from the clinical projects and diverse experiences.

Experience within an Enterprise System

New York University, Division of Nursing, is part of a large enterprise system, comprised of two major medical centers, a home health care agency, and numerous other clinical affiliates including the largest home health care agency in the country. At any one facility, a variety of system projects are in various stages of implementation. The clinical laboratory for the program is both varied and extensive. Students apply their informatics skills to a number of projects in patient care, including case management, quality assurance, and decision support. Working with actual clinical data provides an excellent opportunity for the development of informatics projects. The projects reflect data analysis that support informed decision making in patient outcomes, appropriate interventions, and effectiveness of care.

Students bring to the program varied talents and knowledge of information systems that provide a dimension of richness to the educational experience. Both faculty and students value the opportunity to share and exchange these real life experiences. The large urban setting for the program, with its major medical centers and enterprise systems, provides diverse opportunities for research and clinical projects. One of the more exciting strategies has been to pair nursing informatics students with graduate students in the practitioner programs. These clinical dyads have produced innovative projects including the development of a research project to monitor patients at home with interactive web-based education and communication resources.

What is emerging from these experiences is a model that enhances the learning and knowledge of all involved. Within the context of society today, information technology and informatics have many unexplored avenues for investigation and development. The challenge is to encourage and support innovation for students, faculty, and practitioners as we are swept into the next information wave.

Future Plans

Experience with the program thus far has presented a number of challenges and opportunities. With the rapid expansion of enrolled students, clinical placements will prove to be an issue. Since the program is evaluated both formatively and summatively, changes and revisions on clinical content and course projects will be revised accordingly. The first cohort of students graduated in May of 2000. Thus far, five of the seven graduating students have found employment in informatics positions.

The development of clinical dyads will expand in subsequent semesters. This will involve nursing informatics students pairing up with graduate student nurse practitioners for a specific clinical project. This collaborative model will allow for the clinical specialist to incorporate an understanding of informatics in everyday practice and will promote the informatics skills and knowledge of the informatics nurse. Since we have a number of nurse-run clinics, this will be a value-added benefit for the clinical settings.

SUMMARY

In the past, informatics has been associated with acquiring basic computer skills and knowledge of generic software. As the specialty is articulated, differentiated, and researched, the body of knowledge on the graduate level is becoming more clearly defined. The management of systems and information as it applies to nursing information and knowledge within the context of patient care is the domain of informatics. The potential for the representation and discovery of nursing knowledge within the context of clinical practice is both exciting and possible. The rapid advances in information technology, the availability of information in flexible, retrievable formats, and the need for faculty, students, and nurses to manage large amounts of data and information have driven this shift. Collaboration with other disciplines within health care informatics, the incorporation of experienced clinical informaticists in curriculum design, and the utilization of "real life" clinical projects in an education model are imperative to the success of an informatics program.

The capability and ease of use of technology as well as the changes in health care delivery will be the catalyst in the leveling of the traditional boundaries of education, and informatics will pave the way for the new models. As we reach a "critical mass" of informatics nurse specialists, we will experience an exponential growth of opportunities for nurses practicing in this area. This growth will converge with the rapid deployment of systems in health care that are poised to transform the business of the health care industry.

REFERENCES

AACN (1998). Essentials of baccalaureate education for professional nursing practice. Washington, D.C.: American Association of Colleges of Nursing.

American Nurses Association (1994). *Scope of practice for nursing informatics.* Washington, DC: American Nurses Publishing.

American Nurses Association (1995). *Nursing informatics standards of practice*. Washington, DC: American Nurses Publishing.

AMIA, Nursing Informatics Working Group. Available: URL: *http://amia-niwg.org.*

AMIA Spring Conference (1999). Health Informatics Education. Chicago.

ANCC data on credential nurse practitioners. Telephone communication with Tina Todd of ANCC. September 10, 1999.

Arnold, J. (1996). Nursing informatics educational needs. *Computers in Nursing, 14*(6), 333–339.

Brennan, P. (1995). Patient satisfaction and normative decision theory. *Journal of the Medical Informatics Association, 2*(4), 250–259.

Brennan, P., Lorenson, P., & Ruland, C. (1997). Decision support for assessing patient preferences for geriatric care. In U. Gerdin, M. Tallberg, & P. Wainright (Eds.) *Nursing informatics: The impact of nursing knowledge on health care informatics* (pp. 296–299). Amsterdam: IOM Press.

Carty, B. (1994). The protean nature of the nurse informaticist. *Nursing and Health Care, 15*(4), 174–177.

Carty, B., & Phillip, E. (In Press). The nursing curriculum in the information age. In V. Saba. & K. McCormick. (Eds.). *Essentials of Computers for Nurses: Informatics for the New Millennium.* McGraw-Hill. NY.

Carty, B., & Rosenfeld, P. (1998). From computer technology to information technology: Findings from a national study of nursing education. *Computers in Nursing, 16*(5), 259–265.

Daly, J., Button, P., Prophit, C., Clarke, M., & Androwich, J. (1997). Nursing interventions classification implementation issues in five sites. *Computers in Nursing, 15*(1), 23–29.

Employment Projections. Department of Labor (1999). [On-Line] Available: *http://stats.bls.gov.*

Gassert, C. (1998). The challenge of meeting patients' needs with a national nursing agenda. *Journal of Medical Informatics Association, 5*(3), 263–268.

Staggers, N., Gassert, C., & Curran. C. (in press). Informatics at Four Levels of Practice. *Journal of Nursing and Education.*

Goossen, W., et al. (1998). A comparison of nursing minimal data sets (1998). *Journal of Medical Informatics Association, 4*(2), 152–163.

Graves J., & Corcoran-Perry, S. (1989). The study of nursing informatics. *Image Journal of Nursing Scholarship, 21*(4).

Graves, J., et al. (1995). Description of a graduate program in clinical nursing informatics. *Computers in Nursing, 13*(2), 60–69.

Heller, B., Romano, C., Moray, L., & Gassert, C. (1989). The implementation of the first graduate program in nursing infromatics: A special follow-up report. *Computers in Nursing,* 7(5), 209–213.

Henry, S., & Mead, C. (1997). Nursing classification systems: Necessary but not sufficient for representing "What Nurses Do." For inclusion in computer-based patient record systems. *Journal of Medical Informatics Association,* 4(3), 222–232.

Henry, S., Warren, J., Lange, L., Button, P. (1998). A review of major nursing vocabularies and the extent to which they have the characteristics required for implementation in computer-based systems. *Journal of the Medical Informatics Association,* 5(4), 321–328.

Kelly, K. (1999). New rules for the new economy. Penguin, New York.

Mass, M., Johnson, M., & Mooched, S. (1996). Classifying nursing-sensitive patient outcomes. *Image: Journal of Nursing Scholarship,* 28(4), 295–301.

McCloskey, J. C., & Bulechek, G. M. (1996). *Nursing Interventions Classification* (2nd ed.). St. Louis: C. V. Mosby.

McCormick, K. (1994). Toward standard classification schemes for nursing language: Recommendations of the American Nurses Association Steering Committee on databases to support clinical practice. *Journal of Medical Informatics Association,* 1(6), 421–427.

National Advisory Council on Nurse Education and Practice (1997). A National Informatics Agenda for Nursing Education. Department HRSA. Washington, D.C.

Nursing Informatics Education Programs (1999). [On-Line] Available: *http://amia-niwg.org.*

Ozbolt, J. (1996). From minimum data to maximum impact: Using clinical data to strengthen patient care. *Advanced Practice Nursing Quarterly,* 1(4), 62–69.

Patel, V., & Kaufman, D. (1998). Medical informatics and the science of cognition. *Journal of American Medical Informatics Association,* 5(6), 493–501.

Ribbons, R. (1998). The use of computers as cognitive tools to facilitate higher order thinking skills in nurse education. *Computers in Nursing,* 16(4), 223–228.

Rogers, E. (1995). *Diffusion of innovations* (4th ed.). New York: Free Press.

Saba, V. K. (1992). The classification of home health care nursing: Diagnoses and interventions. *Caring Magazine,* 11(3), 50–56.

Turley, J. (1996). Toward a model of nursing informatics. *Image: Journal of Nursing Scholarship,* 28(4), 309–313.

5

Nursing Informatics: Career Opportunities

Diana Willson, Ginger C. Bjornstad,
John P. Lussier, Susan Matney,
Susanne Miller, Nancy C. Nelson,
Mig Neiswanger, Karen Pinto,
and Cheryl Bagley Thompson

Nurses who receive additional education in the field of informatics are well prepared to enter the job market. As health care organizations attempt to position and leverage themselves within an increasingly competitive marketplace, they are recognizing that a key success factor will be their ability to gather, manage, and utilize information (Lange, 1997; Lorenzi, Gardner, Pryor, & Stead, 1995). The recent

The authors gratefully acknowledge the assistance of the following in the preparation of this paper: Roger B. Buxton, M.S., R.N., Urban Central Region Hospital Director, Nursing Information Systems, Salt Lake City, Utah; Susan Harada, B.S., R.N., 3M Health Information Systems, Salt Lake City, Utah; Rita Snyder-Halpern, Ph.D., R.N., C., C.N.A.A., Associate Professor, Clinical Informatics, University of Utah College of Nursing, Salt Lake City, Utah; Vickie Johnsen, M.S., R.N., Doctoral Candidate, Associate Professor at Brigham Young University, Provo, Utah; Patricia H. Robinson, B.S., Technical Writer, Intermountain Health Care, Salt Lake City, Utah; Julia Rossi, M.S., R.N, Electronic Reference Information Specialist, Intermountain Health Care, Salt Lake City, Utah; Roger Reeves, M.S., R.N., C., Clinical System Analyst/R.N., St. Vincint Hospital, Santa Fe, New Mexico; Brenda Rosebrock, B.S.N., Clinical System Analyst/R.N., St. Vincint Hospital, Santa Fe, New Mexico; Nancy G. Stetson, B.S.N., M.A., R.N., F.H.I.M.S.S., previous consultant for Superior Consultant and Hamilton.HMC; Holly G. Walker, M.S., R.N., Account Executive for vendor of clinical software.

health care initiatives of developing, implementing, and evaluating evidence-based practice guidelines, early intervention and illness prevention programs, and population health and wellness programs while effectively managing costs, all require the extensive and efficient management of data and information. Nursing informaticists who bring with them the knowledge of computer science, information science, and nursing science (American Nurses Association 1994; Graves & Corcoran-Perry, 1996) are being hired by health care organizations who recognize the strategic need for such skilled professionals.

New roles for nursing informaticists are constantly evolving. Informatics roles may encompass any phase of the systems development life cycle: theory formulation, design, development, sales and marketing, selection, testing, implementation, user education and support, maintenance, evaluation, and ongoing enhancements. Other informatics roles can include positions in administration, academics, research, project management, or consulting (American Nurses Association, 1994; Anderson, 1992; Canavan, 1996; Hersher, 1985, 1988; Lange, 1997; McAlindon, 1997; Simpson, 1998). The broad scope of practice for nursing informatics combined with the rapidly expanding body of health care knowledge and the explosion of information technology, makes specialization within the field of informatics increasingly necessary (McAlindon 1997).

The purpose of this chapter is to list and describe some of the many career opportunities available to nursing informaticists. The authors used their own experiences, literature review, and interviews with colleagues to compile the information about the various jobs. The list is not meant to be exhaustive. As new informatics roles evolve, nurses in these new positions find themselves defining the role and creating their own job title and job description. In addition, each organization may define the informatics role and assign responsibilities to meet its unique needs (Anderson, 1992; Lange, 1997; McAlindon, 1997). Minimum requirements for nursing informatics jobs are also changing as nurses with informatics education and experience are increasingly available to fill the positions.

Each of the following career opportunities contains the following subsections: 1) job description that is a brief description of the job and the job responsibilities, 2) job requirements relating to education, experience, interpersonal qualities, and skill sets, 3) the usual setting or physical location of the nursing informaticist, and 4) other possible job titles for this role. Job responsibilities, job requirements, and setting may vary widely depending on the organization. The salary ranges also vary enormously depending on the size of the organization, geographic location, specific job responsibilities and requirements, and years of required education or experience of the informaticist. The authors found salary ranges were generally from $40,000 to $90,000 per year which is similar to other published information (Healthcare Information Management Systems Society 1999). Any notable salary differences or salary calculations are included in the discussions below.

NURSING INFORMATION SYSTEMS COORDINATOR (NIS COORDINATOR)

Job Description

While the job opportunities for nurse informaticists are expanding, the hospital-based setting still represents a large number of nursing informatics positions (Lange, 1997; Rosen & Routon, 1998). Typically, the major job responsibilities of the NIS Coordinator are to coordinate the analysis, design, development, planning, testing, training, implementation, maintenance, support, and evaluation of both existing and future hospital clinical information systems. This is an enormous list of job responsibilities and one that parallels the scope of practice for nursing informatics (American Nurses Association, 1994). While the NIS Coordinator's job responsibilities may be related to nursing applications only, more commonly the NIS Coordinator will also be responsible for many or all of the clinical applications used within the hospital.

The NIS Coordinator serves as a resource to all clinical application system users and troubleshoots with clinicians on a day-to-day basis regarding problems or issues with clinical applications. An effective NIS Coordinator empowers and facilitates users to make decisions, manage applications, and improve information management processes and procedures. Additional job responsibilities may include: the responsibility for re-engineering manual clinical processes into electronic processes for nursing units; coordinating all aspects of user support; and, coordinating the processing and follow-up of requests for modifications and enhancements from users affected by the system.

Job responsibilities for the NIS Coordinator also may include developing training materials and providing computer education on existing and new clinical applications education to all existing and new employees. NIS Coordinators may be asked to work with management and users to conduct studies and analyses of requirements for small, medium, and large-scale integrated systems involving data collection, storage, processing, and retrieval. Keeping up-to-date on trends in nursing practice, hospital policy and procedures, new technologies, and informatics are also frequently specified as job responsibilities for the NIS Coordinator.

Participation in quality improvement teams as well as performing periodic quality checks and improvement projects to assure that the functions of the clinical applications are being performed in an error-free fashion may be responsibilities of the NIS Coordinator. The NIS Coordinator may also create and maintain security files and may assist authorized users in creating the necessary reports, data searches, and information extracts from the information systems.

A common theme seen in NIS Coordinator job descriptions is the responsibility for the coordination of activities related to the information system(s). This coordination may be among nursing departments, the information systems department, and all other hospital departments. The NIS Coordinator may also be asked to coordinate and collaborate with regional, enterprise, or other facility representatives as well as outside consultants and company representatives in the planning, development, testing, implementation, revision, and management of clinical applications. Working with others in collaborative and multidisciplinary work groups is a common theme identified by the NIS Coordinators (Rosen & Routon, 1998). The NIS Coordinator has a significant role as a liaison to represent nursing's unique needs to the Information Systems Department and other departments. The challenge for the NIS Coordinator is to demonstrate an understanding of the needs of clinicians while representing the IS issues at the same time.

Job Requirements

NIS Coordinator positions usually require a minimum of a bachelor's degree in nursing, a current RN license, and several years of clinical nursing experience. The range of requisite computer experience varies greatly among the different position descriptions. Some descriptions state the need for competency in DOS, Windows, and word processing or other PC applications, and previous work with a hospital clinical system while others are more stringent requiring systems analysis, programming languages, and previous experience in areas such as Novell, TCP/IP, and UNIX. Additional skills include oral and written communication skills, ability to maintain good customer relations, technical writing and documentation skills, analysis and problem solving skills, proven interpersonal skills, experience in education of the adult learner, and project management skills. Nursing informatics certification is not a requirement for most informatics positions but is often listed as a preference along with master's preparation in nursing informatics.

Setting

The setting for most NIS Coordinator positions is within the confines of the hospital campus. Some coordinators are located off campus with the data processing department but spend a large portion of their time inside the hospital interacting with users. Some coordinators have responsibilities at more than one hospital site and maintain offices at each facility.

The reporting relationship for this position varies between a direct report to the Information Systems (IS) department, the Nursing Department, or a joint report. Maintaining a strong relationship with the nursing department, regardless of the reporting structure, is essential to the success of the candidate in this position.

Other Possible Job Titles

There are numerous job titles used to describe this position. NIS Coordinator is probably the most recognized and long-standing title. Clinical Information Systems (CIS) Coordinator reflects the move in many facilities to a more multidisciplinary approach. Systems Analyst, Clinical Informatics Analyst, and Clinical Systems Analyst are also used.

CLINICAL INFORMATICS SPECIALIST

Job Description

The job description for a clinical informatics specialist is similar to that of an NIS Coordinator. The major differences are that the Clinical Informatics Specialist is physically located in a corporate office of a large organization and the responsibilities are to the whole organization, not just a single hospital or facility. In addition to the general job responsibilities of the NIS Coordinator, the Clinical Informatics Specialist participates in the organization's strategic planning for information systems development or acquisition, provides the informatics perspective to committees across the organization, maintains a detailed understanding and working knowledge of the organization's information systems, and participates in research projects, presentations, and publications.

The Clinical Informatics Specialist is often considered an "internal consultant." In support of that role are the following job responsibilities: maintaining membership on, or consultation to, committees, work groups, or task forces as needed to communicate and facilitate the ongoing progress of the development, implementation, and revision of clinical information systems; maintaining up-to-date knowledge of trends and advances in the field of nursing and informatics, as well as new developments in hardware and software technology; and, maintaining up-to-date knowledge of nursing practices, regulatory requirements, management and health care issues and trends, and the legal implications of the clinical information systems.

Job Requirements

The minimal requirements include: a bachelor's degree in a health care field or computer information systems; 1 year of clinical health care experience; an understanding and demonstrated knowledge in computers, clinical heath care, and information systems; and, a demonstrated ability to productively manage multiple broad projects at the same time. The preferred requirements are a master's degree in health care informatics, 3 years of clinical health care experience, 3 year's experience as a systems analyst and project manager, 2 years of applicable computer experience in LAN/WAN, PC Client-Server technologies, familiarity with the company's information systems, and formal training in a programming language, systems analysis, and project management.

Setting

The Clinical Informatics Specialist is usually located at an organization's corporate office, but may also be located within a hospital setting.

Other Possible Job Titles

Information Systems Project Leader or Systems Analyst may also be used to describe this role.

DIRECTOR OF NURSING INFORMATICS

Job Description

The Director of Nursing Informatics provides leadership and strategic direction in the development and implementation of the organization's clinical information systems. This executive level position provides guidance to the organization's management team regarding the effective use of information technologies to meet the organization's strategic and operational goals (Lange, 1997). The Director of Nursing Informatics provides leadership during the organization's selection and acquisition of clinical software, internal development of clinical software, implementation and roll-out of existing software, and effective clinical use of the software.

The Director of Nursing Informatics works with established documentation committees to guide their charting from paper to the computer and to re-engineer associated workflow processes, directs evaluation of documentation, and directs the development of new and alternative methods of documentation support.

Quality improvement activities may be an additional job responsibility of the Director of Nursing Informatics. The Director of Nursing Informatics may participate, develop, or guide quality improvement initiatives based on the changing needs of patient populations and the health care environment.

It is important for the Director of Nursing Informatics to keep current about issues and trends in nursing, health care (Lange, 1997), regulatory requirements, and new technologies and their potential applications to health care. The Director of Nursing Informatics position is similar to that of the Clinical Informatics Specialist, but differs in that it is an administrative role as opposed to an "internal consultant" role.

Job Requirements

Minimum requirements are a bachelor's degree in nursing with 5 years experience in direct patient care. Also required are strong technical, clinical, and leadership skills as well as skills in communication, strategic planning, and project management. A master's or doctoral degree in nursing, health care informatics, or related field is preferred. Strong skills in collaboration and negotiation are also helpful for the position (Lange, 1997).

Setting

The Director of Nursing Informatics may be located within a large hospital or at the corporate offices of a health care organization. Service Line Managers, Vice-Presidents of Clinical Services, or Nursing Directors may assume the role of the Director of Nursing Informatics in smaller organizations or those with less computerization in the clinical areas.

APPLICATION SPECIALIST

Job Description

An Application Specialist is responsible for all aspects of implementation for a specific application or a set of applications. Typically, a nursing informaticist would be assigned to "nursing applications" such as charting, medication charting, and care plans although they may also be assigned to other clinical applications. Responsibilities include conducting a systems analysis prior to installing a new application, working with clinicians to re-engineer workflow processes in anticipation of the new software application, training clinical staff to use the applications, coordinating the installation, and coordinating the subsequent user support after installation (Hersher, 1988). An additional responsibility is the ongoing communication with users after implementation for purposes of receiving and evaluating reported bugs and suggested enhancements or modifications of the software.

Job Requirements

Minimum requirements are a bachelor's degree in nursing with clinical experience and knowledge of the systems development life cycle. Written and verbal communication skills, detail oriented, and project management skills are required. A master's degree in nursing or related clinical area is preferred.

Setting

An Application Specialist may be located at the corporate office of a large health care organization, or a vendor of clinical software may also hire for this position. Travel is necessary.

Other Possible Job Titles

The job may also be called Clinical Application Specialist, CIS Coordinator, Installation Coordinator, Systems Engineer, Systems Analyst, Clinical Engineer, Clinical Analyst, or Clinical Implementation Specialist.

ELECTRONIC REFERENCE INFORMATION SPECIALIST

Job Description

The Electronic Reference Information (ERI) Specialist is responsible for utilizing software tools and technologies to make clinical standards and reference information available to clinicians in an electronic format. The ERI Specialist is responsible for participating in the organization's committees that are developing clinical standards and reference materials, educating and advising the committee members as to the issues related to electronic references, and providing guidance as to the physical preparation of the documents that are to be put "on-line."

The ERI Specialist is to become proficient in the functionality of the software tools and is to design electronic documents utilizing informatics theories and current literature about the creation of on-line text references.

On-line text management software is constantly evolving as are web-based technologies. The ERI Specialist must keep up-to-date on the changes in technologies, the availability of commercial clinical reference materials, trends in health care related to practice guide-lines, and legal issues related to utilizing published materials in an electronic format.

Job Requirements

The minimum requirements include: a bachelor's degree in a health-related field, strong computer experience and skills, and effective communication and writing skills. A master's degree in health care informatics is preferred as are previous experience with text man-agement software and project management experience.

Setting

An ERI Specialist may be employed by a large department in a hos-pital, a health care organization, or a vendor.

Other Possible Job Titles

No other job titles are known.

MEDICAL VOCABULARY ENGINEER

Job Description

The job responsibilities include creating, coordinating, implement-ing, maintaining, and evaluating vocabulary for a health data dictio-nary. The Medical Vocabulary Engineer works with end users, clinicians, and software developers to collect lists of terms to be used in clinical software, checks for synonyms and redundancy in submit-ted terms, clarifies the meaning of ambiguous terms, and makes addi-tions and corrections to the vocabulary using appropriate editor/browser tools. Additional responsibilities include optimizing the use of coded vocabulary in clinical applications, placing terms into the appropriate domains and hierarchies to support clinical decision support applications, testing software and associated vocabulary, and training others regarding the structure and possible uses of the data dictionary.

The Medical Vocabulary Engineer must work closely with clinicians, analysts, information systems, and other "customers" to insure vocabulary creation meets the needs of development. The liaison role is important for promoting positive relations with all involved in the vocabulary projects.

Job Requirements

The minimum requirements for a Medical Vocabulary Engineer are a bachelor's degree in health care, health information management, informatics, or medical technology. The ability to use word filters, spread sheets, databases, and word processors is required as is an intimate knowledge of the terms used in medicine. Experience in an inpatient or outpatient clinical setting is strongly recommended.

Setting

The Medical Vocabulary Engineer may be employed at the corporate office of a health care organization or, the position may be with a vendor of clinical software.

Other Possible Job Titles

Systems Analyst or Systems Engineer may be other job titles.

SCREEN DESIGNER AND DEVELOPER

Job Description

A Screen Designer and Developer participates in the analysis, design, development, implementation, and support of applications to meet the data, information, and knowledge needs of clinicians. Historically, programmers were hired to develop software, but with the introduction of new software development tools or "wizards," informaticists are being hired to lead, coordinate, and do both the design and development of clinical software applications.

Job responsibilities for the Screen Designer and Developer

include: meeting with clinical users to understand their data and information needs, using existing tools to design and create data input screens and reports, testing the completed application, and assisting with training the users.

Job Requirements

A bachelor's degree in a health care field or computer information systems is required as is 1-year health care experience and 2 years experience as a project manager or systems analyst. Excellent communication skills, interpersonal relations, and organizational skills are also required. The preferred qualifications are a master's degree in health care informatics, 3 years health care experience, and formal training in a programming language, systems analysis, and project management.

Setting

The Screen Designer and Developer may be employed by a vendor of clinical software or by a large health care organization.

Other Possible Job Titles

Clinical System Architect, Engineer/Analyst, and Informatics Nurse Specialist are other possible job titles.

CLINICAL RESEARCH RN

Job Description

The Clinical Research RN coordinates projects for a specific hospital unit/division or for a project funded by grant monies. This includes coordinating with physicians, nurses, and other clinical staff who will be caring for the research patients. The Clinical Research RN works with the clinical investigators to develop proposals, collect and analyze data, and submit results of the work for review and possible publication.

Job responsibilities include: participating in the development of clinical paths or guidelines; identifying the data needed to monitor clinical interventions and patient outcomes; developing and/or managing the research databases; and, participating in the design, development, implementation, and evaluation of computerized data collection and reporting tools (Lange, 1997).

Typically, the Clinical Research RN is a skilled clinician and, as such, will be able to identify clinical processes and decisions that could be assisted by computerization (Lange, 1997). The Clinical Research RN also assists with clinical training and supervision of staff participating in clinical improvement projects. It is important that the Clinical Research RN maintain up-to-date knowledge of trends in nursing, informatics, and health care in order to promote optimal standards of patient care.

The Clinical Research RN reviews project proposals, manuscripts, and research policies and procedures. In addition, the Clinical Research RN assists with the development and preparation for analysis distribution, and when appropriate, publication.

Job Requirements

The Clinical Research RN must be a registered nurse with three years of direct patient care. Basic computer skills are also required. Informatics experience and/or education is preferred.

Setting

The Clinical Research RN may work at the unit level of a hospital, a division of a hospital, or for a health care organization.

Other Possible Job Titles

Research Analyst and Critical Care Unit (or other specific unit) Clinical Research RN are other possible titles.

DATABASE COORDINATOR

Job Description

The Database Coordinator is responsible for creating, coordinating, and maintaining clinical databases within the organization and assuring the database's compatibility with national databases. This position trains data collectors, oversees the quality of the data collection, oversees the timeliness of the data submission, and provides technical support for personnel responsible for the analysis of the data. In addition, the Database Coordinator is responsible for designing and developing reports used for quality improvement, utilization, and financial analysis.

Other responsibilities include working with individuals and teams to design, create, test, and implement tools for data collection, reporting, and interpretation.

Job Requirements

Minimum requirements are a master's degree in informatics, statistics, or a health-related field with 2 years of relevant health care experience. The Database Coordinator must have an in-depth knowledge of desktop and/or mainframe computer use, with particular emphasis in relational database applications. Additional requirements include: experience in the use of desktop database, spreadsheet, and statistical software; statistical skills including experimental design and descriptive statistics; and, effective communication and leadership skills. A registered nurse is preferred as is the knowledge of Total Quality Management and Clinical Quality Improvement theories.

Setting

The setting may be within a large hospital department, a hospital, or at the corporate offices of a health care organization.

Other Possible Job Titles

The Database Coordinator may also be known as a Data Systems Manager, Systems Administrator, Clinical Analyst, or Systems Analyst.

HEALTH CARE QUALITY IMPROVEMENT AND OUTCOMES MANAGER

Job Description

The Health Care Quality Improvement and Outcomes Manager works as a member of a core team responsible for leading, coordinating, and supporting information management, clinical informatics, decision support, health care quality improvement, and outcomes management across the organization. The person in this position works with others in the organization on the creation and implementation of processes and programs designed to meet operational and patient care objectives that cross facilities, and strengthen the degree of integration and cohesiveness between the facilities, between providers, and between facilities and providers. This includes facilitating collaboration and partnering with physicians for the development of clinical guidelines, interdisciplinary care paths, utilization management, development of interdisciplinary outcome indicators, quality reporting of clinical practice and outcome-based delivery models, and identification of best practices.

The Health Care Quality Improvement and Outcomes Manager will assist in the development and execution of an infrastructure that utilizes information management, sound analytical techniques, and research design methodology, concurrent and retrospective decision support, clinical practice guidelines, and disease management as mechanisms for achieving health care quality improvement and improved outcomes. An additional responsibility is to collaborate with people from information systems, utilization review, managed care, financial administration, and others in the utilization of multiple information systems and development of large databases of clinical and financial outcome indicators. Goals include facilitating presentation of outcomes analyses, trends, and finance reports to clinical and administrative teams in support of continuously evaluating system improvements and provision of patient-centered care.

Job responsibilities also include: conducting and presenting research relevant to health care informatics, health care quality improvement, and outcomes management endeavors to physicians, leadership, management, and governing boards. The Health Care Quality Improvement and Outcomes Manager may be asked to contribute to and draft papers on health care informatics, health care quality improvement, and outcomes management for journal submission.

Job Requirements

Minimum requirements include a bachelor's degree in nursing, 5 years clinical experience and a master's degree in health care informatics, health care administration, or business administration. A minimum of 5 years of health care administrative experience and demonstrated experience in health care informatics, quality improvement or outcomes management is required as is a knowledge of basic principles of epidemiology, biostatistics, and research. Additionally, a working knowledge of DRG, ICD-9-CM, CPT 4 codes, and medical cost accounting is required. Database management, project management, and experience in a relational on-line analytical query tool is also required. Desired skills include skills in teaching, communication, negotiation, project management, leadership, and business acumen.

Setting

The setting may be within a large hospital department, a hospital, or at the corporate offices of a health care organization.

Other Possible Job Titles

In some organizations, Directors of Care Management may be asked to assume the role of the Health Care Quality Improvement and Outcomes Manager.

KNOWLEDGE ENGINEER

Job Description

A Knowledge Engineer is responsible for designing and developing both the knowledge and rules for knowledge applications to be used in the design of expert health care systems (Anderson, 1992). The main focus of the job is information handling relevant to nurses, health care professionals, or other clients, and incorporating medical knowledge into a context and format that is comprehensible by the consumer and able to be manipulated by the computer. The Knowledge Engineer collaborates with clinical experts to elicit knowledge, rules, relationships, heuristics, and decision-making strategies (Anderson, 1992). Then, the Knowledge Engineer uses literature sources to document and analyze health care data and logic and collaborates with software engineers to design and test expert system inference engines.

Other responsibilities include: planning and organization of information content; medical information writing; mapping and compiling using development tools; knowledge engineering; and, editing, testing, and evaluating software and training manuals.

Job Requirements

A current RN license is required. A bachelor or master's degree in nursing is preferred as is experience in a variety of clinical areas. Informatics or computer experience or education is recommended.

Setting

Employment is usually with a vendor or, possibly, with a large health care organization.

Other Possible Job Titles

Expert Systems Analyst is another possible job title.

PRODUCT MANAGER

Job Description

A Product Manager is considered the "product expert" for a business unit, an application, a set of applications, or an entire software package. The primary job responsibility is for over-all product performance including some or all of the following: product content, pricing, positioning, packaging, promotion, cost, competitive analysis, and auditing the product's internal and external performance through its life cycle.

The Product Manager must regularly visit customers to understand job workflow, environment, and business problems and must use creativity and product knowledge to understand and propose products that could be solved by the business unit's current products or enhancements. In addition to visiting customers, the Product Manager must also visit noncustomer sites to understand how problems are solved in their working environment and to gather a comprehensive understanding of functions, features, strengths, and weaknesses of competitive products.

Job responsibilities include proposing solutions to the prospective users' problems through a "market requirements document." The Product Manager documents product functional specifications, while working closely with product development on technical issues included in the document and prioritizes features and functions in upcoming releases, using input from market research and other departments within the business unit. An additional responsibility is to develop and maintain the product's "roadmap" by working closely with all affected departments within the organization to ensure a reliable, predictable, complete, and timely product release (Hersher, 1988).

Participation in trade shows and product demonstrations may be required as might working with the Marketing Department to ensure that all necessary collateral materials, advertisements, public relations, and competitive analyses are implemented. The Product Manager tracks the sales process, follows the sale or loss of sale with a complete win/loss analysis, and uses the win/loss information in the product planning process.

Job Requirements

The minimum requirements are a bachelor's degree and 2 to 5 years of experience with a health care products company or 2 to 5 years of clinical experience. In addition, the job requires superior communication skills, public speaking skills, a "can-do" attitude, good judgment and decision-making skills, the ability to manage multiple projects, and the ability to use creativity and innovative thinking skills to solve business problems observed while working with customers and prospective customers. A master's degree is preferred as is strategic, business, and product planning experience. Travel is usually required.

Setting

The Product Manager is usually employed by a vendor of clinical software.

Other Possible Job Titles

No other job titles are known.

PRODUCT MARKETING SPECIALIST

Job Description

A Product Marketing Specialist is a product or application expert who provides support for the sales staff and provides technical explanations and product demonstrations to the client (Anderson, 1992; Hersher, 1988). Job responsibilities include visiting and interviewing prospective customers to identify requirements and focus areas, working closely with sales and product management, and providing support for the proposal process. In addition, the Product Marketing Specialist coordinates scheduling, planning, and organizing for the demonstrations and provides product demonstrations to support sales efforts.

Job Requirements

The minimum requirements are excellent communication skills, presentation skills, and the ability to handle stress and complex situations confidently. Usually considerable travel is required. A registered nurse is often preferred as is the knowledge of one or more health care software modules.

Setting

The Product Marketing Specialist is employed by a vendor. However, so much travel is required that the person in this position may not have a physical office, but rather a "virtual office" consisting of a laptop computer and modem.

Other Possible Job Titles

A Clinical Product Specialist or Clinical Application Specialist are other possible job titles.

ACCOUNT EXECUTIVE

Job Description

The Account Executive identifies and qualifies potential purchasers of software systems and supporting technologies, and serves as the main marketing and sales contact for organizations within an assigned territory or specifically assigned accounts. The Account Executive coordinates all activities up to and including contract execution.

Job responsibilities for an Account Executive include territory analysis, making contact and introductions with potential customers, follow-up calls, and regular correspondence with prospects. The Account Executive conducts site visits to develop a needs analysis of the client organization and its goals, coordinates the strategic development of marketing planning and activity execution, and leads the implementation team in discussions with the client about project planning and phasing. An Account Executive must be knowledgeable about the business imperatives that health care organizations face with respect to Federal regulatory requirements, third party payer issues, and clinical information surrounding best practice initiatives and outcomes discussions. In addition, the Account Executive must maintain knowledge about competitors' product offerings and sales performance in the territory. Travel requirements are significant, and can indeed frequently translate to a 100% commitment to time on the road.

Sales may offer significant financial benefits, but there are inherent demands that contribute to the challenging nature of this role. Understanding the client and the ever-shifting market are extremely time-intensive; however, the breadth and depth of nurses' experience in the health care arena lay an excellent foundation for success in the sales role. Combined with formal and practical informatics experience and ongoing study of shifting business office issues, nurses are well-prepared to engage executives and clinicians throughout the continuum of health care enterprises.

Job Requirements

The minimum requirements vary, but usually require: a bachelor's degree; a background in computer science or information systems; experience in health care, marketing clinical system software; experience in managing teams; and, the ability to travel and work remotely up to 80%–100% of the time. The Account Executive must be able to build and maintain strong relationships with clients, and be perceived as a knowledgeable and credible resource. Skills in problem solving and responding rapidly to change are essential. A key requirement is the ability to close a sale (Hersher, 1988). Success is measured by the ability to meet assigned quotas.

Setting

The Account Executive is employed by a vendor but due to the extensive amount of travel, may have a virtual office working remotely from the home or area of travel. Considering the amount of data and information that needs to be exchanged in order to conduct business, the Account Executive requires intensive dedicated support by the employer to enable connectivity and problem resolution.

Other Possible Job Titles

The Account Executive may also be known as a Sales Manager, Regional Sales Manager, Marketing Specialist, or Director of Sales.

Salary Information

Salaries vary widely among vendors. Base salaries are usually defined upon the Account Executive's experience and track history in sales. The major financial incentives are commissions paid for signed agreements. The commission structure also varies between vendors: some offer a flat percentage for agreements signed; others structure the commission around incremental increases per dollars signed within annual quota expectations.

CONSULTANT

Job Description

Consultants may be employed by a consulting company or may be self-employed as an independent consultant. Typically, consultants are hired to do one of several jobs: 1) assist with strategic planning (Hersher, 1988); 2) conduct a systems analysis and readiness assessment to assist the client with the many steps in choosing a clinical information system; 3) assist the client in the initial implementation of an information system; 4) assist the client in the further implementation of an information system within the organization; 5) conduct cost-benefit analysis

(Hersher, 1988); or 6) troubleshoot and develop a corrective action plan for information system implementation failures. Organizations who hire consultants frequently do so to meet the immediate need for specific expertise on a short-term project (Simpson, 1998).

Consulting firms have traditionally been focused on the inpatient setting. As outpatient and ambulatory settings have become more common, the firms have had to make that change too. Smaller consulting firms have started to become niche players in the changing arenas of health care.

Consultants spend considerable amounts of time with their clients in conducting systems analyses and interviews with all the individuals involved with the project. Consultants report to the administrator, steering committee, or project manager, who hired them for the specific task. When employed within a consulting firm, the consultant also reports to the Account Manager who, in turn, reports to one of the principals or partners in the firm.

After the data are collected, consultants analyze and summarize the findings and make recommendations. In addition, the experienced consultant identifies additional needs and works with the customer to obtain additional consulting opportunities.

It is important for consultants to scope out the job and to identify the objectives, deliverables, and timeline in the contract. Often, a preliminary meeting will be required to determine the exact nature of the consultation and to ensure that the consultant's expertise is a good match for the job. When the contract is created with a consulting company, the Consulant on site needs to know the scope, deliverables, and timeline. The Consultant will need to renegotiate contract details if other issues, or new issues, arise which are not covered by the contract but the hiring party wants addressed.

Job Requirements

Minimal educational requirements vary from a bachelor's degree to doctoral degree with 3 to 5 years of clinical experience. Experience and/or education in informatics is preferred. Desired skills include: flexibility, ability to prioritize, verbal and written communication skills, conflict resolution (facilitation and negotiation), and presentation skills. Additional skills include analytical problem solving, ability to work independently, creativity, assertiveness, high frustration tolerance, and giving the appearance of credibility (Anderson, 1992; Hersher, 1988). Knowledge of organizational behavior, particularly political and power structures, and skill in determining organizational decision making processes are important for the Consultant. In addition, the Consultant should have experience in word processing, spreadsheet, and presentation applications to facilitate data management and reporting responsibilities. A background in both qualitative and quantitative data collection and management techniques is also helpful.

Setting

Independent consultants are contracted as needed. Employed consultants may have one or more clients they are working with. The settings vary, but generally are with some form of health care organization.

Salary Information

The salary varies widely. Independent consultants bill per job and typically charge the client anywhere from $75–200/hour, plus expenses. Fees are negotiable and are specifically outlined in the contract (hourly fee for "X" weeks and "X" hours/week). Consultants employed by firms may may earn a salary of $65,000, up to $300,000 for the partner level. In this case, the consulting firm invoices the client for "billable" hours at a rate of $140–180/hour, plus expenses. There are firms that have employees that function in a similar manner as Independent Consultants. The firms pay the employee an hourly wage (around $40/hour) when they are contracted with a client, but there is no pay when the individual is between clients.

Other Possible Job Titles

Senior System Consultant, Clinical Informatics Consultant, Project Manager are other possible job titles.

NURSING INFORMATICS INSTRUCTOR

Job Description

The role of the informaticist in a faculty position involves meeting the teaching, research, and service missions of the institution. The proportion of effort spent on each of these components depends upon the type of institution. Faculty located at research universities will have a higher expectation of research and other scholarly activities than individuals at other universities. In addition, some institutions encourage faculty to maintain a practice component to their role.

Teaching is the primary function of most faculty members. The courses taught depend upon the programs offered at the institution. Faculty at universities offering an undergraduate, masters, or doctoral program in informatics usually will teach courses in informatics. Faculty at institutions offering only one or two courses, or a track in informatics may be assigned to other courses such as research, depending upon needs of the institution. Informatics faculty also are responsible for supervising student thesis and dissertation work.

Scholarly activities of informatics can be varied. Informatics scholars may be involved in research activities investigating the impact of various components of computerized systems. However, efforts directed at systems analysis, systems design, and systems implementation also may be considered scholarly activities.

The service role of an informatics faculty member can become quite time consuming. Faculty are expected to serve on college and university committees, as well as to maintain an active presence in the community. Most faculty members are expected to be active in at least one national organization such as the American Medical Informatics Association.

In addition to the three traditional roles of teaching, research, and service, informatics faculty may be expected to maintain a "clinical" practice. Faculty may be asked to assist in systems life cycle activities for the academic unit or affiliated clinical settings.

Job Requirements

Required educational preparation varies across institutions and level of education. Faculty are generally required to have a master's degree within the field of nursing. A doctoral degree usually is preferred (if not required) and may be in any field related to the individual's teaching responsibilities.

Salary Information

Salaries for informatics faculty are consistent with salaries for other faculty members within the same institution. Faculty salaries vary widely depending upon whether they are clinical or tenure track faculty, size of the university, area of the country, number of months in their contract (9 months versus 12 months), degree of administrative responsibility, rank, and years experience.

Other Possible Job Titles

Job titles vary depending on rank. Possible titles are Instructor, Associate Professor, Assistant Professor, and Professor.

THE FUTURE OF NURSING INFORMATICS CAREERS

Career opportunities for nursing informaticists are evolving to fill the ever-increasing information management needs of health care organizations. Health care organizations are hiring informaticists at all levels in the organization: from the unit level to the executive level (Lange 1997). While most informatics positions continue to be with hospitals and health care organizations, home care, long-term care, occupational medicine, and other related health care entities will be looking for informaticists as they begin to computerize (Anderson, 1992). Nursing informaticists will have unlimited opportunities in health care as managers of information and technology (McAlindon, 1997).

It is predicted that changes in health care delivery systems will be driven by two groups: knowledgeable and computer-literate patients who insist on more information and more involvement in their own health; and, "technology-savvy" health professionals who see how these new tools can be used to provide better care (Gates, 1999). The Internet, telecommunications, monitoring devices that download information to a PC or modem, and implantable diagnostic and treatment devices are new technologies that will have a tremendous impact on how clinicians interact with patients and deliver care. Informaticists who understand clinical needs and can visualize how emerging technologies can meet the needs efficiently and cost-effectively will be in high demand.

The future for nursing informaticists is bright. Career opportunities are evolving and multiplying rapidly and will continue to do so well into the future.

REFERENCES

American Nurses Association (1994). *The scope of practice for nursing informatics.* Washington, D.C.: American Nurses Publishing.

Anderson, B. L. (1992). Nursing informatics: Career opportunities inside and out. *Computers in Nursing, 10*(4), 165–170.

Canavan, K. (1996). New technologies propel nursing profession forward: Nursing informatics offers limitless opportunites. *The American Nurse, 28*(8), 1–3.

Gates, B. (1999). *Business @ the speed of thought: Using a digital nervous system.* New York, New York: Warner Book, Inc.

Graves, J. R., & Corcoran-Perry, S. (1996). The study of nursing informatics. *Holistic Nursing Practice, 11*(1), 15–24.

Healthcare Information and Management Systems Society (1999). *1998 HIMSS Annual Compensation Survey.* [Cited June 30, 1999]. Available *http://www.himss.org/himss-member-binaries/compsearch.*

Hersher, B. S. (1988). Careers for nurses in health care information systems. In M. J. Ball, K. J. Hannah, U. G. Jelger, & H. Peterson (Eds.), *Nursing Informatics: Where Caring and Technology Meet.* New York: Springer-Verlag.

Hersher, B. S. (1985). The job search and information systems opportunities for nurses. *Nursing Clinics of North America, 20*(3), 585–594.

Lange, L. L. (1997). Informatics nurse specialist: Roles in health care organizations. *Nursing Administration Quarterly, 21*(3), 1–10.

Lorenzi, N. M., Gardner, R. M., Pryor, T. A., & Stead, W. W. (1995). Medical informatics: The key to an organization's place in the new health care environment. *Journal of American Medical Informatics Association, 2*(6), 391–392.

McAlindon, M. N. (1997). Nurse informaticists: Who are they, what do they do, and what challenges do they face? In J. C. McCloskey & H. K. Grace (Eds.), *Current Issues in Nursing.* St. Louis, MO: Mosby.

Rosen, E. L., & Routon, C. M. (1998). American nursing informatics association role survey. *Computers in Nursing, 16*(3), 171–175.

Simpson, R. L. (1998). Making the move from nurse to nursing informatics consultant. *Nursing Management, 29*(5), 22–23.

6

Precepting Informatics Students: Issues and Perspectives

Diana Willson, Ginger C. Bjornstad,
John P. Lussier, Susan Matney,
Susanne Miller, Nancy C. Nelson,
Mig Neiswanger, Karen Pinto,
and Cheryl Bagley Thompson

An important part of nursing informatics education is the preceptorship experience, or the period of time when the student has an opportunity to apply previously studied theory in a "real life" environment. This can be an exciting and rewarding time for the students, as well as for their preceptors—the people who are involved in supervising the student through the experience. However, as with all educational endeavors, careful planning is required to ensure success.

The purpose of this chapter is to describe issues and perspectives related to precepting nursing informatics students. The chapter describes the roles and responsibilities of the student, preceptor, and faculty in the precepting experience, possible drawbacks or limitations of a preceptorship program, advantages of a preceptorship program, and examples of student experiences. Tools designed to assist in the planning and implementation of a preceptorship program are provided.

The authors gratefully acknowledge the assistance of Patricia H. Robinson, B.S., Technical Writer of Intermountain Health Care, Salt Lake City, Utah in the preparation of this paper.

The authors have a wide variety of experiences related to the preceptor experience: all are nursing informaticists, some have been students in a nursing informatics program, some have been preceptors for nursing informatics students, some have been both student and preceptor, and one is a faculty member who has been involved in the design of a preceptorship program for nursing informatics students.

PRECEPTORSHIP DEFINED

For purposes of this chapter, preceptors are defined as experts or specialists in a field who, for a set period of time, provide guidance and supervision to students who have been assigned to them through an academic program. Preceptorship experiences are offered to students through at least two different types of courses. In the first type of course, the preceptorship experience is not a separate course, but rather exists as a part of a course designed to teach specific concepts (Schoener & Garrett, 1996). An example of this type of preceptorship experience is a decision support course that includes a preceptorship component.

The second type of course, called a "practicum," is a school or college course designed specifically as a preceptorship experience. Practicums can serve many purposes. One purpose is to have the practicum serve as an introduction to a specialty field or a role. Many beginning graduate informatics students could benefit from a practicum designed to introduce the role of an informaticist and the various job opportunities available in the field.

Often, however, practicums are designed as a "capstone" experience. Capstone practicums are usually tailored to the student's interests, strengths, or weaknesses and are usually offered late in the curriculum. They are designed to allow students to apply theory to practice in a supervised, yet real life environment.

Whether a separate course, or not, preceptorship experiences are a valuable part of both the baccalaureate and graduate level educational process. An introduction to nursing informatics practicum would be effective for baccalaureate students interested in pursuing an advanced degree in informatics. However, because of the extensive amount of basic nursing knowledge and practical experience involved in baccalaureate education, the authors believe that preceptorship experiences in informatics should be limited to those students who are returning for a baccalaureate degree after having worked as a registered nurse for at least 2 years.

To be successful, any type of preceptorship program requires careful planning and close coordination among the three people involved: the student, the preceptor, and the faculty. An effective triad can be formed if the roles and responsibilities of each member are clarified and understood at the start of the preceptorship experience.

ROLES AND RESPONSIBILITIES OF THE PRECEPTORSHIP TRIAD

Student Role and Responsibilities

The preceptorship experience should be an exciting and rewarding time for the nursing informatics student. This is the student's chance to put into practice the theory learned in school and to have the opportunity to "see it, do it, and feel good about it." The nursing informatics student must play an active role in the preceptorship process and there are a variety of actions that the student can do to enrich the preceptorship experience. By the end of the preceptorship, the student should gain knowledge in areas of interest and experience or at least familiarity with concepts where he/she is not strong, but are integral to any position as an informaticist. And, the student should begin to have feelings of empowerment, confidence, competence, and satisfaction (Hayes & Harrell, 1994).

To ensure a successful preceptorship experience, it is important that students take responsibility for their own learning. The student needs to communicate to the preceptor about goals and desired experiences. A student's goals should incorporate course goals but should also include personal goals in areas of special interest or in areas of perceived weaknesses (Hayes, 1994).

The student should arrange to meet the potential preceptor prior to the preceptorship program. The initial meeting is the time for the student to assess the preceptor for compatibility and to discuss with the preceptor their goals and the feasibility of meeting these goals during the preceptorship experience. If the student has any concerns about the preceptor or the ability to meet the goals with the preceptor, the student should discuss them with faculty (Hayes, 1994).

At the start of the preceptorship program, the student and preceptor should develop a plan to meet the goals of the student. This plan will serve as the template for the learning opportunities for the student. The student is responsible for working with the preceptor's schedule to participate in as many learning opportunities as possible. In addition, the student needs to be inquisitive and on the lookout for additional learning experiences including observation of the routine, daily activities of the preceptor. The student should volunteer to assist with any project on which the preceptor is working and should anticipate additional tasks or functions that might be helpful to the preceptor or project. Additionally, the student should look for opportunities to share his/her own specialized skills or knowledge with the preceptor.

Periodically, the student needs to monitor the progress against the stated goals. If concerns arise with the lack of progress or other issues with the experience, the student should share them with both the faculty and preceptor. The student should also elicit feedback from the preceptor on a regular basis. Throughout the preceptorship experience, communication is of utmost importance. Both the student and preceptor must know how to reach one another in case of scheduling changes.

Finally, the student must understand the confidential nature of the experiences and of the data and information to which they are exposed. Students may be familiar with confidentiality related to patients or staff members. However, they may be less familiar with the proprietary nature of corporate policies and clinical information system details and the need to maintain confidentiality of this material also. Students may have permission to discuss details of their preceptorship experiences within the confines of the organization and during conferences with faculty and other students. However, students should be reminded frequently that confidential information must not be disclosed outside of the classroom or clinical setting.

Preceptor Role and Responsibilities

The purpose of the preceptor role in nursing education is to introduce the student to a specific informatics job position, provide a socialization experience related to that role, and to provide guidance, supervision, and support while the student applies learned theory in a real life setting (Bain, 1996; Brennan & Williams, 1993; Dibert & Goldenberg, 1995; Hayes, 1994; Hayes & Harrell, 1994; Kersbergen & Hrobsky, 1996; Letizia & Jennrich, 1998; Myrick & Barrett, 1994).

Faculty assess numerous qualifications when looking for potential preceptors. Among the qualifications are the preceptors' interest in precepting, their availability to participate, and the presence and variety of learning opportunities that the preceptor can provide for the student. Preceptor professional qualifications include informatics experience, peer respect, participation in professional issues, positive leadership role modeling qualities, and interest in professional growth. The faculty will consider communication style and skills, teaching skills, critical thinking skills, and personality traits when selecting preceptors (deBlois, 1991; Hartline, 1993; Hayes, 1994; Hayes & Harrell, 1994; Letizia & Jennrich, 1998; Schoener & Garrett, 1996; Yonge, Krahn, Trojan, & Reid, 1997). While nursing informaticists are most often considered as potential preceptors, the authors don't believe that being a nurse or an informaticist should be a requirement. Other skilled professionals may be able to provide learning experiences that meet the unique learning needs of some students.

Before deciding to participate, the potential preceptor should clarify with the faculty the goals of the class, the expected weekly time commitment, the duration of the preceptorship experience, the amount of responsibility the preceptor will have for evaluating the student, and the expected frequency of communication with the faculty (Byrd, Hood, & Youtsey, 1997). The potential preceptor should realistically evaluate the current job responsibilities and workload to see if additional preceptor responsibilities can be accommodated. In addition, the potential preceptor may need to seek permission to precept students from their immediate supervisor. Finally, if the potential preceptor feels the need for instruction or review of preceptor skills, faculty should be consulted as to how best to meet those needs.

During the preceptorship experience, the preceptor should plan and set aside specific times to meet with the student. The preceptor should discuss with the student the role, job responsibilities, daily routine, current and future projects, and organizational or political issues. The preceptor has the responsibility to assist students in finding learning opportunities to meet course and student goals. Both the preceptor and student should be constantly on the lookout for potential learning opportunities for the student. The preceptor should assess which projects and tasks within the facility could involve the student and whether the student should observe or actively participate in the projects. The broad scope of roles or job types in informatics makes it improbable that one preceptor can provide a student with all the experiences desired. However, the preceptor may be able to temporarily place the student with other professionals who can provide additional learning experiences for the student.

The preceptor should assist the student in integrating and interpreting the various experiences of the student. Sometimes a debriefing is necessary after a particularly lively meeting or encounter that the student witnesses. The preceptor can explain to the student the history, personalities, and political agendas that led to the series of events or decisions. Feedback to the student should be provided routinely and especially after the student has participated in a project (Hayes & Harrell, 1994).

Ultimately, the preceptor should be prepared to assist the faculty in the final evaluation of the student. In addition, the faculty will want feedback about the experience, information on if and when the preceptor is interested in repeating the precepting experience, and suggestions for improving the experience for all involved (Hayes, 1994).

Faculty Role and Responsibilities

Successful precepting experiences are the result of careful planning and guidance of the supervising faculty (Schoener & Garrett, 1996; Usher, Nolan, Reser, Owens, & Tollefson, 1999). Students should not be sent to the clinical arena without careful orientation of both the student and the preceptor. Faculty members are responsible for careful selection of sites, matching of students and preceptors, orientation of students and preceptors and evaluation of the experience from both the preceptor and student perspective (Dibert & Goldenberg, 1995; Myrick & Barrett, 1994; Usher, et al., 1999).

Site selection is an important component of the faculty role. Faculty must select a site that will offer the student a set of experiences that will match the objectives of the course and the personal objectives of the student. The faculty also must assure that individuals at the site are capable and willing to supervise the student.

Student preceptor matching is an additional component of the faculty role. Not all students are appropriate to match with a given site or preceptor. Faculty should be familiar with the students' background so as not to place them at a site that will merely offer experiences that are repetitive of previous experiences (Yonge et al., 1997). Faculty also should consider the individuals in the student/preceptor dyad when making assignments. Placing an individual in a student role with someone to whom they are related or for whom they work may create difficulties for both parties.

Faculty are responsible for orientation of students and preceptors. Students need to be informed of course expectations and specific site requirements. Some institutions may require that students acquire a hospital ID and computer password, attend an orientation session, and/or sign a confidentiality and nondisclosure statement prior to working with a preceptor. Faculty are expected to help students to understand what they may or may not do as part of their role as a student. Faculty also are responsible for informing students of methods for dealing with conflict in the clinical setting. The student should be made comfortable with discussing institution or preceptor issues with the faculty member.

Faculty members are responsible for orientation of preceptors to their role (Byrd, Hood, & Youtsey, 1997; deBlois, 1991; Hayes, 1994; Schoener & Garrett, 1996). Even individuals that have been a preceptor previously will need to know the specific objectives of the new course. For new preceptors, a face-to-face meeting is suggested. However, a phone call is usually sufficient for experienced preceptors. The faculty member needs to be aware of time constraints placed upon the preceptor and be willing to provide orientation as needed.

Informal group meetings are an enjoyable way to provide individuals with preceptor orientation. A luncheon, hosted by the faculty, can provide an opportunity for faculty to provide information in an expedient manner. This approach also allows newer preceptors to learn from conversation with more experienced preceptors.

Faculty have responsibility for continuing oversight throughout the preceptorship process. Faculty need to check in with the preceptor as well as the student to see that activities are progressing as planned and to offer assistance in dealing with any problems that arise. Faculty must also assure that the learning objectives are being met and that mechanisms are in place to deal with problems as they occur, whether they stem from student or preceptor difficulties. Finally, the faculty play an important role in helping the student understand, integrate, and generalize their experiences (Hayes & Harrell, 1994; Schoener & Garrett, 1996; Yonge et al., 1997).

Evaluation is the final component of the faculty role (Schoener & Garrett, 1996). The faculty should have a specific plan for course evaluation. Evaluation techniques can include verbal or written communication with the preceptor. The faculty may elect to use a formal evaluation form or to conduct an informal verbal evaluation. Faculty also should provide students the opportunity to evaluate the experience as well as the preceptor and environment. Finally, faculty should bring closure with the preceptor by providing feedback about the student's perception of the learning experiences, asking the preceptor about their own experiences, exploring with the preceptor means of improving the preceptorship program in the future, and asking if the preceptor would like to participate again. Faculty should maintain regular correspondence with past and future preceptors for purposes of keeping them updated as to course changes, informed as to when their services may be requested again, and enthusiastic about participating in the preceptorship experience.

PRACTICAL TOOLS TO FACILITATE THE PRECEPTING EXPERIENCE

The authors have developed two tools that they believe will facilitate the precepting experience. The first tool is called the "Checklist for a Successful Preceptorship Experience" (Table 6.1). The checklist details the numerous tasks for which the student, preceptor, and faculty should be responsible in order to ensure success. The checklist is meant to assist faculty in the development of a preceptorship program. Further, if the checklist is shared with students and potential preceptors, the roles and responsibilities of each member of the preceptorship experience should be made clearer.

The second tool is called the "Checklist of Learning Opportunities" (Table 6.2). The purpose of the checklist is to facilitate understanding regarding the personal goals of the student and the potential learning opportunities that could be provided by the preceptor. The checklist should be completed by both students and potential preceptors and given to the faculty. The faculty will use the checklist to help accomplish the important task of matching student to preceptor.

TABLE 6.1 Checklist for a Successful Preceptorship Experience

✓	Task/responsibility	Comments
	*** Faculty Check List***	
	Select potential preceptors based on pre-determined criteria • Availability of preceptor • Opportunities for students at preceptor site • Interest/willingness in being a preceptor • Informatics experience • Peer respect • Reputation in the community • Effective communication style/skills • Effective teaching skills • Critical thinking skills • Decision-making abilities • Positive leadership/role modeling qualities/skills • Awareness/participation in professional issues • Personality traits (patience, warmth, humor, empathy, etc.) • Previous experience with precepting • Interest in professional growth • May want to consider other disciplines besides nursing	
	Invite potential preceptors to participate in the program • Clarify time commitment • Clarify expectations • Explain role of preceptor • Discuss skills needed by the preceptor • Discuss preceptor responsibilities • Allow potential preceptor to say "no" • Explain the next steps the preceptor should expect	

TABLE 6.1 *(continued)*

✓	Task/responsibility	Comments
	Ask potential preceptors and students to complete the "Checklist of Learning Opportunities"	
	Match students with preceptors based on their responses to the "Checklist of Learning Opportunities." Also consider a student's past experiences and personalities of both the preceptor and student.	
	Address any institutional policies (contracts, confidentiality, and non-disclosure agreements, logons/passwords for students)	
	Assist the preceptor in any necessary training (role clarification, principles of adult education, teaching methodology, learning theory, feedback concepts, assessment of learning needs, learning contract, evaluation theory, and methods). Assistance can be in the form of reading recommendations, informal education, and ongoing consultation.	
	Communicate available days/times for phone calls, consultations, additional meetings.	
	Provide the preceptor with written information which includes: • Criteria used to grade the student • Information about who evaluates and grades the student • Preceptor responsibilities • Student hours required • Length of time of the program • Scheduled meeting times with faculty	

TABLE 6.1 *(continued)*

✓	Task/responsibility	Comments
	Provide the student with written information which includes: • Criteria that will be used to grade them • Information about who will evaluate and grade them • Student responsibilities • Student hours required (per week, month, quarter, semester, etc.) • Length of time of the program (month, quarter, semester, etc.) • Scheduled meeting times (with faculty)	
	Consult with preceptor at the end of the course. *Discuss:* • The success in meeting student goals • What the most valuable experiences/ lessons learned by the student were • Possible improvements or changes that could occur to improve the experience *Determine:* • How did the preceptor feel about the experience? • What impact (positive or negative) did the experience have on the preceptor? • What could the faculty or student do to improve the experience? • Would the preceptor be willing to participate again? *Provide feedback to the preceptor:* • Student perceptions • Strengths of the experience • Possible areas of improvement	

TABLE 6.1 *(continued)*

✓	Task/responsibility	Comments
	Maintain contact at each semester/quarter/ year with past preceptors. Inform them as to whether their services will be asked for again. Keep preceptors appraised of changes in the curriculum/program.	
	If feasible, maintain contact with students and evaluate, 1-year post practicum, whether the experience was helpful and relevant, and if there are suggestions for making the experience more helpful.	
	*** Student check list ***	
	Complete the "Checklist of Learning Opportunities."	
	Provide resume or curriculum vitae to faculty for sharing with preceptor. Keep it current.	
	Develop personal objectives/goals desired from the preceptorship program and prioritize them.	
	Meet potential preceptor. • Explain personal goals and ask if they are reasonable and possible. • Assess personality traits and communication style of the potential preceptor. Will compatibility be a problem? Discuss concerns with faculty. • Determine how best to reach the preceptor and at what times.	
	Schedule the first day to meet and spend time with the preceptor.	

TABLE 6.1 *(continued)*

✓	Task/responsibility	Comments
	Take responsibility for own learning • Schedule meeting times with preceptor • Volunteer to assist with projects/tasks preceptor is working on • Anticipate what additional tasks might be helpful to the preceptor and volunteer to do them • Ask for and accept feedback routinely from preceptor • Work with preceptor's schedule to attend/participate in as many learning experiences as possible • Monitor progress against goals	
	Take responsibility to share specialized skills/ knowledge with the preceptor (two-way learning)	
	*** Preceptor task list ***	
	Consult with faculty. Clarify the following: • General goals of the experience for the student • Time commitment involved (per week) • Duration of the preceptorship program (month, quarter, semester, year) • Communication frequency with faculty • Responsibility for evaluating the student (what role does preceptor have)	
	Determine if current job responsibilities and work load will allow for the extra time and effort required to fulfill role of preceptor	
	Examine preceptor skill sets and determine learning needs (role clarification, principles of adult education, teaching methodology, learning theory, feedback concepts, assessment of learning needs, learning contract, evaluation theory, and methods).	

TABLE 6.1 *(continued)*

✓	Task/responsibility	Comments
	Involve faculty if additional education in the role of the preceptor and training related to preceptor skill sets as needed	
	Complete the "Checklist of Learning Opportunities."	
	Provide to faculty contact information (phone numbers, pager numbers, best days and times for making contact)	
	Provide recent resume or curriculum vitae to faculty for sharing with students and other preceptors	
	Meet potential student. • Evaluate student learning goals and determine if they are reasonable and possible given your current job responsibilities. • Assess personality traits and communication style of the potential student. Will compatibility be a problem? • Determine how best to reach the student and at what times.	
	Take responsibility for the following: • Set aside specific times with the student for teaching and role modeling. (Discuss with student your role, job responsibilities, daily routine, current and future projects, organizational/political issues.) • Assist student in finding learning opportunities and experiences. Involve others in the institution/facility who could assist with a specific experience.	

TABLE 6.1 *(continued)*

✓	Task/responsibility	Comments
	• Assess which projects/tasks could involve the student and whether the student should observe only or also participate. • Anticipate what additional tasks might be helpful and ask if the student would be willing to do them. • Ask for and accept feedback routinely from student about the experience and if it is meeting the student's goals. • Provide feedback to the student if student has participated in any tasks/projects. • Assist student in integrating and interpreting experiences. • Assist faculty in final evaluation of student.	
	At end of preceptorship program, communicate with faculty: • Overall impression of the experience • Time commitment involved • Positive (and negative) experiences • What faculty or future students could do to improve the experience • Whether there is interest in being a preceptor again	

The students' completed Checklist of Learning Opportunities should be given to the selected preceptor so that the preceptor will have an understanding of the specific goals of the student and the skills that the student may already possess. The preceptor will use the checklist to plan the learning opportunities for the student. Both students and preceptors must understand that no preceptorship can possibly provide for the students all of the skills and experiences on the checklist. However, by using the tool, the best matching of student needs to precepting possibilities is possible.

TABLE 6.2 Checklist of Learning Opportunities
(To be Completed by Student and Preceptor)

(Indicate what kind of experience is desired or possible and whether the experience is to be observed (Ob) or participated in (Pa), or both. Use the Comments column for details/comments/questions. Students indicate if they have had previous experience (Prev Exp)).

Method Ob Pa	Skill/experience	Comments	Prev exp
	*** New application/function development ***		
	Study phase (initial research into the problem, user meetings)		
	Analysis phase (preliminary work, feasibility assessment, user needs assessment, process flow diagrams, data flow analysis, workflow analysis)		
	Definition phase (general/logical design, modeling, prototyping, data flow diagramming)		
	Project proposal, prioritization, and review process (development, submission, review)		
	Request for proposals (RFP) (development)		
	Review and evaluation of RFPs (vendor review)		
	System/function design (functional specifications, input screens, output reports, user interface, clinical algorithms and alerts)		
	Construction phase (liaison interpreter work with programmers and users)		

TABLE 6.2 *(continued)*

Method Ob Pa		Skill/experience	Comments	Prev exp
		Testing phase (plan and test— acceptance, integration, volume and stress, multiple-site, regression, security/controls, usability, and bug reporting)		
		Training phase (needs assessment, determine type of training, plan, plan training budget, develop materials, conduct training)		
		Implementation phase (plan, project manage, back-out planning)		
		Evaluation phase (evaluate existing, plan for evaluation of new product)		
		*** **Other informatics experiences** ***		
		Data modeling		
		Data or communication standards		
		Network/communications		
		Database design/construction		
		Knowledge engineering		
		Data dictionary work (vocabulary, taxonomies, definitions)		
		Hardware (test, install, set up, evaluate, maintain)		
		Text management skills (Folio, web)		
		Web technologies (develop, test)		
		Ongoing support/maintenance (user rounds, user groups, programmer meetings)		

TABLE 6.2 *(continued)*

Method Ob Pa	Skill/experience	Comments	Prev exp
	System/hospital integration and consistency issues (Y2K, new versions of hardware/software)		
	Regulatory/government requirements (JCAHO, FDA regulations, HCFA regulations)		
	Organizational/political issues (decision process within the organization, organizational chart, "power" people/departments/projects, barriers to projects)		
	Interface (specification, design)		
	Ergonomic issues (mental, physiological, emotional, behavioral)		
	Human-computer interface (assess, design)		
	Software development (programming, "wizard" use)		
	Data warehouse (define data, search, group, report)		
	Care process/care map/clinical algorithm (analyze data needs, design, implement, evaluate)		
	Population/outcome studies (analyze, design, develop, evaluate data)		
	Quality Assurance (define, analyze, evaluate quality indicators)		
	Role socialization ("day in the life of")		

TABLE 6.2 *(continued)*

Method Ob	Pa	Skill/experience	Comments	Prev exp
		*** "Administrative" experiences ***		
		Budget planning (yearly, by product, by department, total I/S budget, training budget for project, overall software training budget for year)		
		Basic health care business functions (accounting, finance, economics, marketing, reimbursement practices)		
		Information needs assessment		
		Information management planning (for department, hospital, corporation)		
		Priority setting (yearly, by department)		
		Customer/consumer relations		
		Meetings (user group, nursing administration, information systems, work groups)		
		Confidentiality, Security issues (policy review, development)		
		Product documentation (specifications manuals, user documentation)		
		Policy making related to computers or use of computers		
		Project management (readiness for change, task estimates, critical path, schedule/Gantt, budget, risk analysis, tool use)		
		Product management (evolution of product, "road map" planning, market analysis, quality markers)		

TABLE 6.2 *(continued)*

Method Ob	Pa	Skill/experience	Comments	Prev exp
		Sales/marketing/promotion of medical software/hardware (product demonstrations, producing sales literature)		
		Contract negotiations		
		Ongoing relationships with vendors		
		Consult/provide expertise (to other disciplines, organizations)		
		*** **Professional experiences** ***		
		Conferences (attend, present)		
		Publications (write, review, critique)		
		Education (teach, attend classes)		
		Networking (meetings with professional colleagues)		
		Professional organizations (plan, attend meetings)		

Projects change and evolve through time and as a result, the preceptor's roles may change. Consequently, the faculty should ask all preceptors, even the experienced ones, to complete a checklist prior to each new matching of students to preceptors.

LIMITATIONS OR DRAWBACKS OF THE PRECEPTORSHIP EXPERIENCE

Limitations from the Student Perspective

Although a preceptorship experience presents many opportunities for students, the experience may at times also present difficulties. Students frequently face challenges in trying to coordinate their schedules with those of the preceptor and the learning opportunities available. Scheduling conflicts are magnified if the student is trying to juggle school with work and family obligations.

Learning opportunities available in preceptorships will vary and this variation may seem to some students inequitable. Variation in learning opportunities is normal and is due to differences among the participating sites, the coincidental timing of the preceptorship with projects at the site, each student's goals and unique strengths and weaknesses, and compatibility between student and preceptor. If a student is concerned about the learning experiences during the preceptorship, the student may find helpful a discussion of the concerns with both the preceptor and the faculty.

Finally, compatibility problems between the preceptor and student may occasionally develop. Conflicts can range from personality clashes to differing perceptions of student readiness to take on certain tasks (Hayes, 1994). Again, any concerns on the part of the student should be discussed with the preceptor and/or faculty.

Limitations from the Preceptor Perspective

While the benefits of being a preceptor are many, drawbacks also exist. The extra time, energy, and resources required of the preceptor are significant (Beauchesne & Howard, 1996; Byrd et al., 1997; Hayes, 1994; Letizia & Jennrich, 1998; Usher et al., 1999; Yonge et al., 1997). The nature of the experience may necessitate having a nursing informatics student with the preceptor for extended periods of time, often requiring the preceptor to alter daily schedules to accommodate the demands of the preceptor role. Days that may have been planned in solitary activities like reading, developing, or editing documents, or similar activities may need to be rescheduled in order to interact with the student.

Preceptors often feel that they have to always be "on stage": always explaining and discussing rationale behind their actions. Explaining the rationale behind each action, task, or decision takes extra time and this can be very draining for the preceptor. Preceptors report that this constant verbalization of otherwise internal and very rote thought processes is the most wearing. Further, time spent explaining takes away from time spent actually working, thus causing anxiety to the preceptor knowing that tasks are waiting to be completed, and that some loss of efficiency to the institution through incidental delay in normal coordination assignments has occurred (Hayes, 1994; Yonge et al., 1997).

Additionally, preceptors may feel that in order to get the student up to speed on a project, they must provide extensive background on a project or explain a group's history to help the student understand why a certain decision was made. When the preceptor cannot take the time to do extensive explaining, the preceptor may be left with a feeling of providing less than optimum experience for the student.

Some preceptors may find that the lack of privacy; having someone shadow you for an entire day, leaves little time for personal activities. The preceptor may feel guilty taking the time to read e-mail or answer phone mail messages, since this is time not spent interacting with the student.

Sometimes, finding a rewarding educational opportunity during the period of time of a preceptorship experience also can be a challenge. While many worthwhile projects may be underway at the institution, the timing may not be right for student involvement. Excellent student experiences occur when the student is able to take on a project from start to finish, but this is rarely possible given a student's time constraints or the fact the projects may already be underway when the student starts the preceptorships. Finding rewarding experiences in some highly technical areas also may be difficult. While the student may have the necessary technical skills, the project may involve a great deal of knowledge of the proprietary system before any independent work can be done and the preceptor rarely has enough time to get the student up to speed in the allotted time of the preceptorship.

Preceptors generally receive little training in precepting skills. Faculty may assume that since the nature of the nursing informaticist is teaching and assessing readiness to learn, a preceptor understands principles of adult education and has conflict resolution skills. However, even the best preceptors may have difficulty providing negative feedback to the student when necessary. Many preceptors have asked for help in these areas (deBlois, 1991; Dibert & Goldenberg, 1995; Hayes, 1994; Letizia & Jennrich, 1998).

Finally, even the best nursing informaticist may not be the best preceptor. Precepting is not for everyone or for everyone all the time (Hayes & Harrell, 1994; Usher et al., 1999). The preceptor needs to carefully consider workload, time commitments, and overall stress level before consenting to participate in each preceptorship experience.

Limitations from the Faculty Perspective

From a faculty perspective, the practicum sometimes creates two students, the preceptee who is trying to understand the new role, and the preceptor who may require guidance or support in the event of problems. Even with experienced preceptors, faculty sometimes find trying to remain in contact with the preceptor very time consuming. This task is more difficult when the preceptor does not have consistent office hours or is not available by phone.

Another challenge is managing students placed in a variety of settings and supervising several asynchronous practicums where the students have spread the practicum over several semesters, several facilities, and/or several preceptors. Similarly, equalizing the experiences for the students can be challenging. Those students placed in highly computerized and progressive facilities may appear to have a much richer experience.

The students often want to discuss their experiences and often focus on those experiences where things could have gone better. Effective faculty can help students to use these stories as a learning experience, discussing what could have been done better, and rationale for the outcome. Additionally, faculty are often challenged with the task of explaining the inconsistencies and differing philosophies that students report across the different facilities. The faculty have to be prepared for anything, as students may bring literally any issues from their practicum. While this can be rewarding, trying to anticipate the questions and issues and to remain well-versed in many areas can be challenging.

ADVANTAGES OF A PRECEPTORSHIP PROGRAM

Advantages from the Student Perspective

Nursing informatics students participating in a preceptorship program have the opportunity to practice the theory learned in school in a supervised, supported, and nonthreatening environment. The preceptorship provides the unique experience to practice skills before actually being employed in the field. The student can observe and participate in projects while being protected from unnecessary stress and conflict and can observe bureaucratic conflicts and frustrations of the everyday world without bearing responsibilities for the problems (Letizia & Jennrich, 1998).

Students will experience enhancement of previous theoretical learning by the application of skills and knowledge to real life situations. The process of trying new skills in a protected and neutral environment should increase the student's self-confidence in trying new and diverse roles, improve problem solving skills, foster independence, and facilitate skill development (Byrd, Hood, & Youtsey, 1997; Hayes & Harrell, 1994; Letizia & Jennrich, 1998; Schoener & Garrett, 1996).

Students, through their preceptors, will participate in collaborative experiences and will meet and associate with a variety of other clinicians and informaticists. Such experiences will be the start of a lifelong benefit of networking among professional peers.

Students will gain an understanding of the role of the nursing informaticist. This is the first step into "role socialization" and the start of the journey from a novice level to an expert level of practice (Benner, 1984; Lewis, 1986). Some students, after completing the preceptorship experience at a facility, are later hired by that facility. When this happens, it is considered a benefit to all concerned: the student has a job in informatics, the facility has hired a well-qualified person, and the school can demonstrate that students are finding jobs after graduation.

Advantages from the Preceptor Perspective

Advantages and benefits also exist for the preceptor, although frequently they are subtle, personal, and individualized. Certainly, one advantage is that discussions between the preceptor and student force the preceptor to examine his/her own knowledge, reflect and evaluate upon his/her own practice, and serve as continuing education and re-education for the preceptor (Bain, 1996; Usher et al., 1999; Yonge et al., 1997).

Preceptors enjoy watching their students develop professionally. Contributing to the profession of nursing and nursing academic programs may increase the preceptor's feelings of self-worth. Preceptors may experience job enrichment and personal and professional growth (Brennan, 1993; Dibert & Goldenberg, 1995; Hayes, 1994; Hayes & Harrell, 1994; Lewis, 1986; Usher et al., 1999; Yonge et al., 1997). As has been the experience of several of the authors, preceptors may decide to pursue graduate level education in informatics after they see those whom they have helped teach flourish professionally.

Improvement and validation of precepting skills in areas of problem solving, leadership, assessing learning needs and styles, planning educational experiences, and evaluating may prove satisfying for the preceptor. Because these same skills are frequently valuable during the course of the preceptor's normal work, the preceptor may receive tangible benefits from the experience (Lewis, 1986; Usher et al., 1999; Yonge et al., 1997).

Precepting provides the satisfying opportunity for the preceptor to network with students, faculty, and other preceptors. Most preceptors find the experience enjoyable, stimulating, and often, quite frankly, fun.

Advantages from the Faculty Perspective

A practicum or preceptorship program allows the faculty to provide individualized learning experiences that will meet the needs of students who enter the program with a wide variety of skills and experiences. Faculty can place students with a preceptor in an environment suited to the students' interests, strengths, and weaknesses.

During the preceptorship experiences, faculty have the opportunity to network with practicing nursing informaticists in a variety of settings. Faculty will directly observe current issues and trends in the field and collect data on their current curriculum in order to update, redesign, and develop their academic programs. The obvious benefit to the faculty is to minimize gaps between theory and practice (Brennan & Williams 1993).

EXAMPLES OF STUDENT PRECEPTORSHIPS

No practical limit exists to the number of projects in which a student can observe and participate in. The only real challenge to an effective experience involves matching the student's timeline and personal and class objectives to the most appropriate ongoing project(s). The following are examples from the authors' precepting experiences.

The examples illustrate some of the keys to a successful preceptorship experience and some of the situations that may lead to a less than optimal experience for the students. While some experiences have proven more rewarding than others, the most successful student experiences have had several factors in common: excellent timing of the preceptorship with the specific project and the ability of the student to have "hands on" experience working on a project.

The first example involved an unusually rapid implementation project. An implementation date for a specialized nursing documentation project was set for late May. A student in a graduate informatics practicum arrived in early March, just in time to be catapulted into the final phases of the project, which included de-bugging, testing, staff training, installation, and support. The student was able to participate in all phases of this process. Once oriented to the project, the student productively assisted in testing and de-bugging the software, including the discovery of programming faults and inconsistencies that the designers and preceptor had not yet recognized. The student was also able to participate in the development of the training tools and the training plan and taught several of the staff training classes. Finally, the student was able to participate in the implementation and support phase of the project, and in fact spent several shifts on the unit providing on-site support to the staff during the initial implementation. The compressed time line of this project fit perfectly with this student's academic schedule to provide a very comprehensive experience.

Another successful preceptor experience occurred when two preceptors working in the same facility had students from the same academic class. The preceptors were about to pilot a new quality monitoring program on an acute care unit and invited the students to jointly participate in the implementation of this project as part of their practicum. The students worked together on an implementation plan, developed training tools, taught classes and provided user support when the program was installed. They developed evaluation criteria for the project and completed the evaluation of the new program after the installation. Based on their evaluation and the success of this pilot project, the program was implemented throughout the facility using their tools and methods. This situation was successful in that the students had the opportunity to use their skills in a real implementation, and they were able to experience, first hand, the realities of working in groups and accommodating the abilities and styles of coworkers.

The least successful preceptorship experiences have occurred when student or course goals have not correlated well with activities at the preceptor site. In these cases, students came to the facility with predetermined and detailed objectives that frequently did not mesh with projects that were ongoing at the facility at that time. This situation often meant that the preceptor had to make up or contrive a project on which the student could work. One example of this occurred when a student in a decision support class needed to find a related project on which to work. While the facility had many ongoing decision support protocols in place, no new projects were underway at the time of the student preceptorship. In order to meet the student's project goals, the preceptor developed a hypothetical project based on a real clinical need. The student designed, built, and "implemented" a prototype strictly within the walls of the computer lab. The student did not have the opportunity to implement the project in the clinical setting with real users, and thereby missed the most important and distinguishing opportunity and purpose of a "real-world" preceptorship program. The authors feel that mismatches such as this one are more apt to occur if the preceptorship experience is directly tied to a specific course in the program, such as decision support, system analysis, or implementation, as opposed to making the preceptor course a separate course within the curriculum.

THE FUTURE OF PRECEPTORSHIP EXPERIENCES IN NURSING INFORMATICS EDUCATION

When graduate nursing informatics education first began, few practicing nursing informaticists were available with whom faculty could place students (Lange, 1997). Therefore, the potential learning opportunities for students were rather limited and faculty found that matching student goals with precepting sites was difficult. Now, however, the potential pool of preceptors is growing rapidly. Students entering nursing informatics programs are now more easily matched with preceptors who can help them meet their educational goals.

This is an exciting time for nursing informatics education. Everyone benefits from the preceptorship experience: students have an opportunity to practice skills learned in school, preceptors find the experience satisfying and rewarding, and faculty can continuously evaluate and improve the educational opportunities for students so they can graduate students well prepared to enter the real world of nursing informatics.

REFERENCES

Bain, L. (1996). Preceptorship: a review of the literature. *Journal of Advanced Nursing, 24*(1), 104–107.

Beauchesne, M. A., & Howard, E. P. (1996). An investigation of the preceptor as potential mentor. *Nurse Practitioner, 21*(3), 155–158.

Benner, P. (1984). *From novice to expert.* Menlo Park, California: Addison-Wesley Publishing Co.

Brennan, A., & Williams, D. (1993). Preceptorship: Is it a workable concept? *Nursing Standard, 7*(52), 34–36.

Byrd, C. Y., Hood, L., & Youtsey, N. (1997). Student and preceptor perceptions of factors in a successful learning partnership. *Journal of Professional Nursing, 13*, 344–351.

deBlois, C. A. (1991). Adult preceptor education: A literature review. *Journal of Nursing Staff Development, 7*(3), 148–150.

Dibert, C., & Goldenberg, D. (1995). Preceptors' perceptions of benefits, rewards, supports and commitment to the preceptor role. *Journal of Advanced Nursing, 21*, 1144–1151.

Hartline, C. (1993). Preceptor selection and evaluation: A tool for educators and managers. *Journal of Nursing Staff Development, 9*(4), 188–192.

Hayes, E. (1994). Helping preceptors mentor the next generation of nurse practitioners. *Nurse Practitioner, 19*(6), 62–66.

Hayes, E., & Harrell, C. (1994). On being a mentor to nurse practitioner students: The preceptor-student relationship. *Nurse Practitioner Forum, 5*(4), 220–226.

Kersbergen, A. L, & Hrobsky, P. E. (1996). Use of clinical map guides in precepted clinical experiences. *Nurse Educator, 21*(6), 19–22.

Lange, L. L. (1997). Informatics nurse specialist: Roles in health care organizations. *Nursing Administration Quarterly, 21*(3), 1–10.

Letizia, M., & Jennrich, J. (1998). A review of preceptorship in undergraduate nursing education: Implications for staff development. *The Journal of Continuing Education in Nursing, 29*(5), 211–216.

Lewis, K. E. (1986). What it takes to be a preceptor. *The Canadian*

Nurse, 82(11), 18–19.

Myrick, F., & Barrett, C. (1994). Selecting clinical preceptors for basic baccalaureate nursing students: A critical issue in clinical teaching. *Journal of Advanced Nursing, 19*, 194–198.

Schoener, L., & Garrett, M. P. (1996). Faculty: The driving force in preceptorship. *Nursing Connections, 9*(3), 37–42.

Usher, K., Nolan, C., Reser, P., Owens, J., & Tollefson, J. (1999). An exploration of the preceptor role: Preceptors' perceptions of benefits, rewards, supports and commitment to the preceptor role. *Journal of Advanced Nursing, 29*(2), 506–514.

Yonge, O., Krahn, L., Trojan, L., & Reid, D. (1997). Through the eyes of the preceptor. *Canadian Journal of Nursing Administration,* Nov–Dec, 65–85.

7

Web-Based Informatics Education: The Duke University Model

Linda Goodwin, Norman McIntyre,
and Kevin Sprecher

The world we have made, as a result of the level of thinking we have done so far creates problems we cannot solve at the same level which we created them.
—Albert Einstein

Teaching as we know it today derives from the great philosophers Aristotle, Plato, and Confucius—and an oral tradition in which interactions of teacher and pupil, master and novice allowed for the transfer of specific facts and information and sowed the seeds of knowledge. Through the ages, as technology has developed, the process of teaching and learning has also evolved. In today's world, however, one can barely remain even with, much less ahead of, the technological wave. Thus a new paradigm of technology-based pedagogy and its application to learning is coming of age.

BACKGROUND AND OVERVIEW

Information doubles approximately every 18 months. Textbooks and other printed matter are often obsolete before they are available to the masses. In the last 5 years alone, many of the worlds' maps have had to be redrawn to reflect dynamic geopolitical realities. Yet information is not knowledge. It is the basis of knowledge, but it is not knowledge in and of itself. Knowledge is the ability to use information in a creative and purposeful way. At the end of the twentieth century, pedagogy remains relatively unchanged from medieval times.

To promote learning and knowledge, the pedagogy of the next millennium must incorporate technologies and define itself anew rather than continuing to deliver old ideas in a bright, high-tech box.

OLD TIMES, NEW TIMES

This chapter addresses all four aspects of the model in Figure 7.1 and describes the main elements that must be considered in explicating fundamentals of technology-based pedagogy.

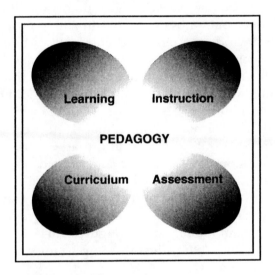

FIGURE 7.1 Pedagogy Model.
With permission: http://www.mllc.org/pedagogy.htm.

In old paradigms, the professor demonstrated mastery or competence on a given topic by professing specific facts, formulas, and other pieces of information to a targeted group of individuals. These individuals are expected to take in these pieces of information, determine their relative value or relevance, and regurgitate on demand. This "tell'em and test'em" format has been shown to be ineffective in promoting real learning. Unfortunately, this is the method that most of the world's learning institutions utilize and the one with which most individuals, both faculty and students, are comfortable.

But new paradigms and pedagogy are emerging with the next millennium, and the challenge for nursing in general, and informatics in particular, is to embrace this new technology-based pedagogy and decide when its use is appropriate and when other more traditional, or yet unexplored new methods are more suitable. There will certainly continue to be content areas and concepts that require personal classroom contact for learning.

This chapter will discuss how Duke University made progress toward an innovative Nursing Informatics program that illustrates the challenges of the new paradigm. Paradigms are either bridges or barriers to change and innovation. It is difficult to propagate change from the outside and even more difficult from within a given paradigm. Despite technology, approaches to teaching and learning have not significantly changed. While the packaging of information has changed from a print-based to an audio-visual medium, the goal is still the dissemination of information, coupled with the ability to regurgitate that information on demand. As we become more techno-centric, this skill will be as antiquated as the buggy whip. According to economist and futurist James Davidson, the economic value of memorization as a skill will fall while the importance of synthesis and creative application of material will rise. Examples of this paradigm shift in Duke's Nursing Informatics program include team projects and domain modeling (see Figures 7.6–7.13), and student portfolio deliverables that reflect this important synthesis and creative application of new learning.

INSTRUCTION: THE NEED FOR BANDWIDTH (BOTH TECHNOLOGICAL AND COGNITIVE)

If we can change the price and performance of bandwidth and long distance, if we can collapse distance and time, something big is going to happen.
—Joseph Nacchio, CEO Qwest Communications

Indeed something big is going to happen and it is happening now in the manifestation of cheaper and faster bandwidth. Cheap fast bandwidth will totally revolutionize learning and pedagogy as we know it today. The ability to transmit large volumes of data in the form of digitized photos and video will no longer be dependent on expensive and/or specialized equipment. Virtual simulations will be enhanced by the ability to mimic responses in real time or with imperceptible delays. But as with most revolutions, the outcomes of change are filtered by existing paradigms and not valued for what they truly represent. This "paradigm blindness" delays and inhibits the realization of benefits from innovation (Brownstein, 1998). Thus mental attitude adjustments and "increased bandwidth" thinking (to adopt that metaphor) will be needed for new paradigms of pedagogy to emerge.

Paradigms represent our mental constructs or the framework of "our" world—the ways we perceive, think, place value and bias. Because our paradigms are often implicit rather than explicit, we rarely lift them up to the light of examination. Rather, we seek to explain that which is new or different in the context of our paradigm. When the explanation derived is congruent with the constructs of our paradigm, we maintain a sense of equilibrium. If, however, the explanation lacks "fit" with the construct, a state of cognitive dissonance is created. As humans tend to seek equilibrium, the dissonance is resolved in one of two ways: either the phenomenon and its explanation are rejected out of hand or they are incorporated into the existing paradigm, creating a shift in perception, values, and beliefs and thus re-establishing equilibrium.

We are at risk of developing paradigm blindness (or at least myopia) if we try to fit the technological revolution and its implications within the context of our current educational paradigms. To plan for the future with what we know now is to lock in preconceived notions, ideas, and misconceptions that will prevent us from exploiting the full spectrum of virtual education. Posting of lecture notes or static textbooks on a web site is not innovation. Rather, it is the repackaging of information from one medium to another. The true outcome of web-based teaching is beyond our comprehension and will be the result of an iterative, evolutionary process shaped by many minds and hands.

> *The problem is never how to get the new innovative thoughts into your mind, but how to get the old ones out.* —Dee Hock, founder and former CEO of Visa

In moving forward to embrace new pedagogy, educators and institutions must pause to examine their own paradigms for higher education. Brownstein (1998) points to a number of assumptions and institutional behaviors at risk for assault by the technological tidal wave bearing down on us:

- Students are viewed as scarce commodities to be competed for.
- The arena of competition local, regional, or national, varies only depending on the reputation of the school.
- High exit barriers, particularly in graduate school, in the form of difficulties in transferring credits, block students from choosing courses from many different schools in a degree program.
- Demographics are the prime mover of student enrollment.

If for any given institution these assumptions are true, then the behavior of the institutions, congruent with its paradigm, is as follows:

- A majority of courses are taught utilizing "tell them, test them" pedagogies by professors providing little more than information.
- The pervasive idea is that Internet teaching is merely the challenge of getting lecture notes and other static information on a web page.
- Little or no attention is paid to the questions of appropriate pedagogies for this new medium.
- The essential facts about what is needed to respond to new challenges are assumed to be knowable, rather than something to be discovered.

Current pedagogies will continue indefinitely. The dominant pedagogy is still what one student colorfully called "tell them and test them." In the old paradigm model, the student is the passive learner and the professor has the information. To be sure, marginal changes such as group work have been introduced into this pedagogy but the primary source of learning in this model is the professor. The focus in the old paradigm is on providing information and not creating knowledge.

Big organizations don't change, they die! —Tom Peters

CURRICULUM: CONCEPTUALIZING ON-LINE NURSING INFORMATICS COURSES

At Duke University, a new program in nursing informatics was first approved, in 1996, through traditional academic and curriculum channels. Courses focused on the developing field of nursing informatics, which combines nursing science, computer science, and information/decision science (ANA, 1994) and examines issues in applying nursing informatics within complex health care organizations and administrative structures. Students were required to have basic prerequisite personal productivity (computer) competencies. Course content was directed toward assisting the student to understand the relationships between the current state of nursing science, health care reform, and complex informatics issues. The courses seemed to lend themselves to the new virtual paradigm of distance learning and web-based instruction. After all, this *is* an informatics specialty immersed in technology, and it made sense to leverage the new program using a technology-based approach.

CURRICULUM: CLINICAL CONTEXT

Development of the Nursing Informatics program was based on the view that informatics knowledge and skills are most effectively applied by experts who are also advanced practitioners in an area of clinical specialization; that is to say, applying the tools appropriately requires expertise in the domain to which the tools are being applied. Duke's faculty believes this expertise is best demonstrated by nurses who have completed graduate education as well as years of advanced clinical experience. Thus the courses are open only to nurses who are completing a post-master's certificate program, or meet experience criteria and are near the completion of their master's degree. Program content focuses on the preparation of advanced practice nurses who can demonstrate knowledge and skills in the development of clinical information systems at all phases of a system's life cycle. Other kinds of programs to educate nurses for informatics work in a variety of other health care arenas (e.g., teaching informatics) are still needed.

A growing issue in Nursing Informatics education is the qualifications and experience of faculty who are teaching courses sometimes incorrectly titled "informatics." Since nursing is a practice discipline, practice experience in Nursing Informatics should be foundational for teaching content in the domain. However, as graduate nursing programs seek to expand and recruit students, it is not uncommon to find that someone with only basic personal computing skills is asked to teach a "Nursing Informatics" course. Many of these faculty are fine academicians but they frequently lack experience with clinical information systems, and they may or may not have experience with instructional technology. Thus the content required to help nurses learn the knowledge and skills needed to use clinical informatics in their own practice, or in positions with vendors or health care agencies, is sadly lacking. A challenge for the new millennium is to help educate our colleagues about the distinctions between teaching computer/technology and (nursing) informatics content.

CURRICULUM: INFORMATICS CONTENT

Duke's Nursing Informatics Program combines a block of on-campus time each semester with web-based content mastery and a clinical residency in which students are placed with mentors to work on real-world projects. Mastery is demonstrated by completing a "take home" quiz at the end of each virtual lecture, and a competency-based and proctored exam is given on campus after completion of two semesters. The general areas of content are listed below.

- *CAMPUS*: Historical Perspectives, Web Design and HTML Authoring, First Principles and Systems Life Cycles, Object Oriented Analysis and Design, Unified Modeling Language (UML), Written Requirements and Problem Domain Modeling, User-Centric Design Methodologies, Emerging Technologies, NI Professionalism, hands-on Technology Labs.
- *WEB (OVER TWO SEMESTERS):* Issues related to health care, nursing, information systems, and ethics, law, regulations, policy, politics, economics, technology, complexity, teamwork, and standards. Theoretical applications of systems, expertise, information processing, diffusion of innovation, change, artificial intelligence, knowledge discovery in databases (KDD), decision support, and quality outcomes.
- *RESIDENCY (THIRD SEMESTER):* The student is placed with a mentor in an area of interest and spends a minimum of 156 contact hours to complete personal and course objectives. The goal of the residency experience is to provide immersion in a real-world project that helps students synthesize their clinical expertise with informatics issues, relevant standards, theories, and technology applications in health care.

CURRICULUM: CONTEXT AND PROCESS

Since distance-based learning brings a new set of problems and opportunities, the curriculum is designed around a student-centric model that is depicted in Figure 7.2. The goals include the creation of a learning environment (culture) that is perceived by students as supportive of their individual learning needs in a caring and collaborative context, while providing organized structure and sound principles of curriculum design to facilitate their optimal learning. Providing a supportive virtual learning culture has turned out to be more difficult than anticipated, and we learned a great deal in the first year that has considerably improved subsequent students' experiences!

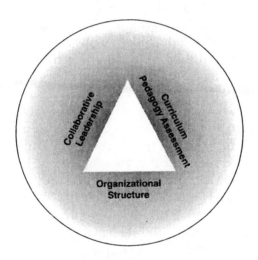

FIGURE 7.2 Student-Centric Model.
With permission: http://www.mllc.org/project.htm.

A student-centric model requires helping students and faculty make the transition from traditional to new paradigms. Duke's program combines 4–5 days on campus with 13 weeks of distance-based instruction. The program offers informatics students access to a new philosophy of teaching and learning that they review before they come to their first campus class. The Web-based information provides a foundation for discussion of core values and what students hope to gain from their academic experience. Thus far, this seems to have facilitated the transition from old to new paradigms of pedagogy. The paragraphs below illustrate the information shared with students as pre-campus preparation for launching into the program. *With permission: (http://www.duke.edu/~goodw010)*

The current state of the world for both kindergarten-through-high school and higher education results in too many students of all ages and in all settings being focused on grades rather than on their learning. Most of us in the United States (and probably around the globe) were trained to sit glued in our chairs taking notes as fast as we could and generating our best guesses at what needed to be memorized for regurgitation on exams and papers. We were lectured by the "Sage on the Stage." But educators' journals are filled with research about how little retention (therefore how little TRUE learning) occurs with this form of teaching. Emerging teaching and learning paradigms are adopting a "Guide on the Side" faculty role. However, faculty who are experts in their field have difficulty giving up their Sage role. Because true learning takes effort and involvement on the part of the learner, the new pedagogy creates a structured learning environment for the student to navigate with assistance. The faculty's role is to provide the structure, the resources, and the environment for learning; this is the most appropriate role for a new learning paradigm. But students who have spent most of their academic careers in old paradigm classrooms sometimes grow frustrated with their "Guide on the Side" and desperately want the "Sage on the Stage" to just tell them what they need to know. This may minimize immediate frustration but it rarely improves true lifelong learning.

Most of us were also raised in competitive learning environments where we tried to out-do our classmates, or resigned ourselves to being inferior when we could not successfully compete. The majority of today's work environments are too complex for isolated employees to be productive with a competitive attitude. Today, employers succeed when they create environments for cooperative teamwork inside the organization, and view their competition as the external marketplace. Internal competition is counterproductive for employees as well as the employer. There is an increasing need for teamwork in the workplace as well as the classroom. Therefore, teaching and learning paradigms MUST promote teamwork and cooperative learning. Since nursing remains a primarily female profession, gender roles and issues complicate the development of authentic teamwork and cooperative learning in the profession. (Playing house with dolls was never a TEAM sport.) But awareness is a good place to begin.

The following 11 points give the "Digest" version of Dukes' Nursing Informatics faculty philosophy, and goals for working with learners of all ages, in all places, and at all times. The *Hitchhiker's Guide to the Galaxy* series, by Douglas Adams (1979) is delightfully silly and recommended reading for students. Page 2 of the Hitchhiker's Guide has the words DON'T PANIC in big bold letters, and instructions to refer to page 2 when in doubt. Duke's Nursing Informatics program has multiple references to "page 2" throughout the courses!

GUIDING PRINCIPLES FOR LEARNING

1. The professor doesn't know ALL the answers . . .
2. Create a community of self-directed learners with a spirit of teamwork and collaboration.
3. Encourage students to identify and act upon their own learning needs.
4. Encourage active learner participation and involvement.
5. Give and share resources, skills, knowledge.
6. Use really current (WWW) reading and resources.
7. Take new risks: go where you've never gone before.
8. NO wimps and NO whiners. There is TOO much to learn, and learning is incompatible with cowardice, whining, and complaining. (Yes, learning takes EFFORT on the learner's part and is sometimes hard . . .)
9. Use creative thinking, critical thinking. Form educated opinions, then defend them.
10. Aim for almost paperless courses . . . (Save trees and help our environment).
11. Make it FUN—learning is easier that way!!

Feedback from students suggests that success has been achieved in all these principles except for paperless courses. Even though electronic versions are provided for most course materials, students still have a tendency to print things and file them in notebooks. The ultimate goal is full-fledged on-line courses in which faculty are active participants in the adoption and diffusion process and give meaning to classes, while students take responsibility for their own learning as well as development of a virtual learning community.

LEARNING AND ASSESSMENT OF LEARNING: SETTING RIGOROUS STANDARDS

From the outset, Duke's Nursing Informatics program has used rigorous standards and expected excellent outcomes of learning. Assessment involves evaluating students' performance with regard to specified core competencies that are based upon, but expanded beyond those of the American Nurses' Association. *Nursing Informatics* is defined by the American Nurses' Association Task Force on the *Scope of Practice for Nursing Informatics* (1994) as a scientific discipline that serves the profession of nursing by supporting the information handling work of other nursing specialties. *Nursing Informatics* is the specialty that integrates nursing science, computer science, and information science in the identification, collection, processing, and storage of data and information to support all levels and all specialties of nursing practice, administration, education, and research. Three levels of competencies have been established for nursing informatics. It is important for nurses to differentiate these levels and fully comprehend the level at which they are prepared to practice. It is also important for students to understand the level at which their academic coursework prepares them to perform.

At the minimum level of competency (ANA, 1994) *all* nurses should be able to identify, collect, and record data relevant to the nursing care of patients. They should be able to analyze and interpret patient and nursing information as part of the planning for and provision of nursing services. Additionally, they should use health care informatics applications for the clinical practice of nursing and implement public and institutional policies related to privacy, confidentiality, and security of information, including patient care information, confidential employer information, and other information gained in the nurse's professional capacity.

At the next level of nursing informatics practice, basic competencies include the development and evaluation of applications, tools, processes, and structures that assist nurses with data and information management. This is the level of competency that is mastered in Duke's Nursing Informatics program. Students are challenged to distinguish generalist from specialist nursing informatics practice, and to strive for specialist practice through lifelong learning and experience.

Many of Duke's Post-Master's Certificate students are able to function at the level of the informatics nurse specialist (INS). An INS has a master's degree in nursing and has taken graduate-level courses in the field of informatics. The INS is prepared to assume roles requiring advanced knowledge of nursing and of informatics. According to the ANA *Scope of Nursing Informatics Practice* (1994), specialists in nursing informatics must be competent in the following areas:

- Design and/or implementation of nursing informatics science and applications to clinical and/or healthcare administrative problems.
- Analysis and evaluation of information requirements for nursing practice.
- Appraisal of computer and information technologies for their applicability to nursing practice.
- Development and teaching of the theory and practice of nursing informatics.
- Consultative practice in the field of nursing informatics.
- Collaboration with other health informatics specialists and other specialists from supporting disciplines in the creation or application of informatics theory and practice for nursing.
- Development of strategies, policies, and procedures for introducing, evaluating, and modifying information technology applied to nursing practice.

The Duke Graduate School of Nursing Informatics curriculum is based upon five pillars of content, competencies, and skills that give advanced practice nurses:

1. hands-on technology skills
2. clinical information systems life cycle and project management experience
3. domain modeling skills
4. broad fundamentals from computer science and information processing theory
5. critical thinking skills needed for informatics research and development.

A checklist (Table 7.1) is used to help students and faculty assess the student's entry level and desired level of competence in a variety of nursing informatics skills.

Examples and more information for learning assessment results are provided later in this chapter. At the end of the Duke Nursing Informatics program, students submit a portfolio that documents their skill level and provides samples (and evidence) of deliverables for competencies, coursework, and residency projects. These portfolios often serve as material for consideration during job interviews and/or promotions. Duke's faculty utilizes the portfolio to evaluate each student for overall program learning, deliverables' quality, and final competency as they complete the program. Portfolios, to date, reflect that innovative Nursing Informatics instruction at Duke has made significant progress toward a new paradigm and pedagogy; we are accomplishing our goals of educating the "next generation" of clinical nursing informatics leaders.

INSTRUCTION: EXPERIMENTS IN INNOVATION

As a pioneering effort to provide techno-centric and distance-based education in nursing as well as informatics, Duke's program developed five main strategies and a particularly innovative new content area in the early years of the program. The new content area came to be labeled "domain modeling" and introduced concepts of object-oriented analysis and design to expert nurses. The hope was that expert nurses could use these object-oriented tools to map the knowledge domain of our profession and help translate that to others, including information systems developers. Innovative instructional strategies, tempered by practical realities, included:

- Content and process delivery via web-based technologies
- Participative learning strategies and assignments
- Required teamwork for assignment completion
- Experiments with pros and cons of synchronous versus asynchronous interaction.

INSTRUCTION: WEB-BASED TECHNOLOGIES

Several different options were tried for web-based instruction, but the method preferred by students employed streaming audio tech-

TABLE 7.1 Competency Checklist Excerpt (Full List Is 6 Pages)

Directions:
If you have no experience with what the competency requires, mark *"clueless"*
If you believe you can begin to perform the competency, but need mentoring, mark *"novice."*
If you believe you can independently and comfortably perform the competency, mark *"proficient."*
If you believe you could provide leadership and mentor others in the competency, mark *"expert."*

Desired competency	Clueless	Novice	Proficient	Expert
Nursing science and skills				
Problem identification (system level)				
Advanced practice critical thinking skills				
Integration of holistic patient perspectives				
Integration of research and practice findings				
Integration of quality improvement concepts				
Integration of patient outcome analysis				
Integration of resource consumption analysis				
Generation of creative solution options				
Integration of teamwork skills				
Therapeutic communication skills				
Research critique and utilization				
Abstractionism skills				
Technical skills: Hardware & software				
Hardware selection, config, install, troubleshooting				
Software selection, config, install, troubleshooting				

TABLE 7.1 *(continued)*				
Desired competency	Clueless	Novice	Proficient	Expert
Word processing (list package/s)				prereq
File management				prereq
E-mail				prereq
Web browsing/ resource mining				prereq
HTML web page development				
Spreadsheet skills (list package/s)				prereq
Database skills (list package/s)				prereq
Presentation skills (list package/s)				prereq
Project Management skills (list package/s)				
Domain Modeling skills (list package/s)				
Clinical info system #1 (list vendor)				
Beyond basic nursing informatics practice:				
Integration of relevant nursing standards and advanced practice expertise				
Systems analysis—domain modeling				
Employment of principles from supporting disciplines				
Project management				
Integration of relevant concepts and standards				
Integration of applied theories				
Computer Science skills:				
Information/Decision Science skills:				

nologies with a combined software approach that uses MS PowerPoint *(http://www.microsoft.com)* slides and RealAudio *(http://www.real.com)* technology. Figure 7.3 shows an example of the student view when they "attend a (web-based) lecture," and both the slide and audio controls appear on the screen. Students navigate through the slides and audio at their own pace, repeat items that need additional work, and stop and start the lecture at their own convenience.

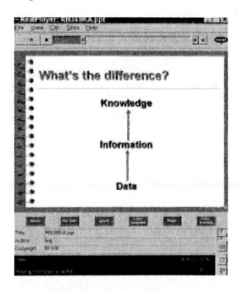

FIGURE 7.3 Sample "Lecture" Screen.

INSTRUCTION: PARTICIPATIVE LEARNING BY DESIGN

When the first-year courses were offered in Duke's program, web-based content required HTML coding and was both tedious and time consuming. By the second year, web-based content was delivered via a Lotus Notes Domino Server *(http://www.lotus.com)* and pre-structured templates for rapid entry of standardized structures, which saved time but also resulted in less flexibility for delivery of content. Synchronous chat primarily used a free software download of ICQ *(http://www.mirabilis.com)* which students used for completing their team assignments, and faculty used for virtual office hours. Synchronous modes of communication also included audio and video conferencing, but not all students had these technologies and bandwidth rendered their use via modem from home not always practical. As the screen in Figure 7.4 shows, an asynchronous on-line seminar was achieved through use of a "forum" structure that used threaded discussion technologies. Student views do not include the "participation, scores, setup" options at the bottom of the screen; these are reserved for faculty use. The "core values" listed as the mission on the forum introduction were compiled by students during their first on-campus weekend.

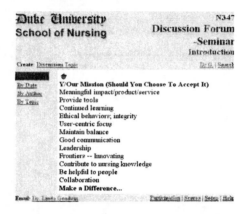

FIGURE 7.4 Forum Discussion Main Screen.

INSTRUCTION: WEB DEVELOPMENT BASICS

One of the assignments students complete during their first on-campus weekend is a web page that provides information to help them get acquainted with other class members. When students are dispersed all over the country (and the world), these web pages help them connect with and remember their virtual classmates. The format is left open and flexible to allow students to experiment and learn at their own pace.

Over the course of the program, students acquire more advanced web development skills and work in teams to generate a health-related web site. Content has ranged from patient education for knee injury and treatment options, genital herpes, and preterm birth symptoms to organizational Internet and Intranet sites. One team chose a content area that would educate consumers about privacy issues and computerized patient records (Figure 7.6).

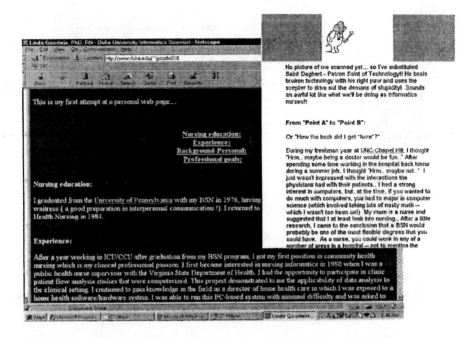

FIGURE 7.5 Sample Screens—First Web Project (Personal Introduction).

LEARNING: VIRTUAL TEAM PROJECTS

Traditional systems analysis, written requirements, and systems specifications have failed to produce the clinical information systems needed by nurses who provide direct care for patients. Under the tutelage of Charles Mead, MD, CEO (CareCentric Solutions, Inc.—Duluth, GA), Duke's Nursing Informatics Program embarked on a pioneering effort to help nursing informaticists learn new skills of abstractionism and domain modeling. Using object-oriented analysis and design and an emerging standardized notation called the Unified Modeling Language (UML), Dr. Mead was instrumental in launching this new content into the nursing informatics curriculum at Duke, and Duke has now been followed by other schools of nursing.

Within the context of advanced practice nursing, the domain modeling and applications developed by Duke's Nursing Informatics students include development of personal digital assistant (PDA) technologies for clinical documentation and outcomes

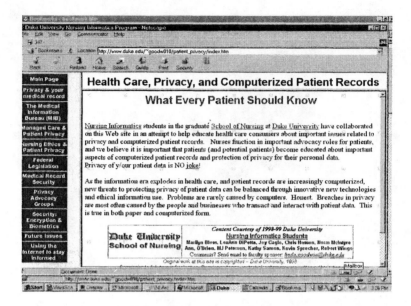

FIGURE 7.6 Sample Screen—Advanced Web Project.

data collection. Domain modeling to understand the needs of the advanced practice nurses who need improved information systems is a difficult task that is best accomplished by nurses who understand the clinical domain and the technology being developed for use within that domain.

Figures 7.8 and 7.9 are a subset of domain modeling deliverables that are embedded within an assignment to develop written requirements for an advanced practice nursing application. Standardized notation with UML (Unified Modeling Language) creates use case models with stick men and elipses that are deceptively simplistic. But when used to interact with developers and end users, they are exceedingly powerful and effective communication tools. The segment of a use case diagram and description, below, illustrates this phenomenon and also provides an example of a virtual team project that is part of the new learning paradigm at Duke University School of Nursing.

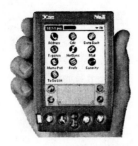

FIGURE 7.7 Palm Pilot—Personal Digital Assistant Technology. *http://www.palm.com/*

EXAMPLE VIRTUAL TEAM PROJECT: USE CASE MODELING

Use Case Analysis (Pain Management Documentation Application)

(Credit and thanks to Marilyn Bloss, R.N., M.S.N. and Ann O'Brien, R.N., M.S.N.—class of 1999)

A use case is defined as an interaction between the system and an actor that results in the fulfillment of a system responsibility that produces a product of value for the actor (Booch, Jocobsen, & Rumbaugh, 1999). At its highest level shown here in Figure 7.8, most nurses and information systems developers will find a use case model a place to begin dialogue about system requirements. A high level use case serves as a focal point to begin the translation process between user requirements and technical development. This translation role is one where nursing informatics roles have historically shined but also annoyed developers by insisting on clinical domain details that were not easily understood by the technical experts. Use case models are visual tools to help with the translation and communication process.

As high level use cases are "de-composed," that is more detail is explicated, the diagrams often become more complicated. "The devil's in the details" is an important fact when developing clinical information systems. The ability to abstract those details to a level where all team members understand the user requirements and technical constraints is an important skill that Duke's program attempts to enhance and improve.

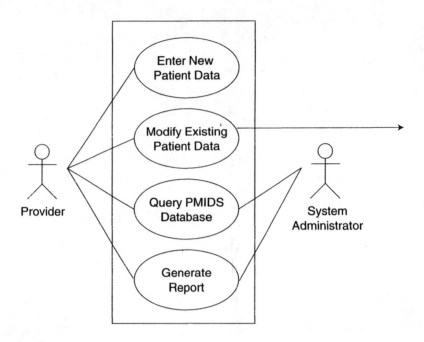

FIGURE 7.8 High Level Use Case Model.

Definitions

(System) Pain Management Information Documentation System (PMIDS): The system which will be used in the Pain Management service at XYZ Big Health Care System to capture data for all patients receiving assessment and treatment of acute and chronic pain. The PMIDS database will be utilized for daily management of PMIDS patients, tracking and trending of PMIDS statistics, pediatric benchmarking, medical/nursing research, patient billing and documentation of advanced nursing practice and outcomes.

(Actor) Provider: The user authorized to enter, modify, transfer, query, and report PMIDS data for a specific patient using the Pendragon Forms Manager *(http://www.webfayre.com)* on the desktop PC and the Pendragon Forms on the PalmPilot *(http://www.palm.com)*. Providers include the PMIDS advanced practice nurse, the attending anesthesiologist, and the anesthesia resident.

Modify Existing patient Data

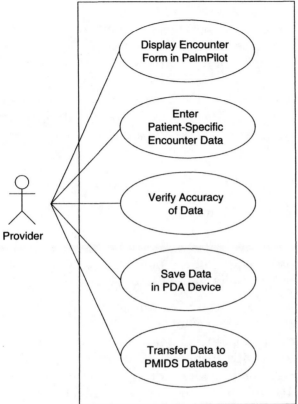

FIGURE 7.9 Use Case Decomposition for One of the High Level Use Cases.

(Actor) System Administrator: The user responsible for updating, modifying, and maintaining the PMIDS system design and database structure. The system administrator has control over the configuration and security of the system and generates aggregate data in the form of reports. Thus, the system administrator also has the capability of performing queries and generating reports of the data in the PMIDS database.

(Use Case) Enter Data: The Use Case in which the provider creates a record for a newly admitted PMIDS patient and enters patient-specific historical information into the PMIDS database.

(Use Case) Modify Existing Patient Data: The Use Case when the provider updates or edits patient-specific data in the PMIDS database.

(Use Case) Query Data: The Use Case when the Actor (provider or system administrator) makes requests to the system for specific and/or aggregate information from the PMIDS database.

(Use Case) Generate Report: The Use Case when the Actor (provider or system administrator) produces standardized and/or specialized reports on patients in the PMIDS database.

Use Case Description #1

Name: Enter New Patient Data

Actor: Provider

Goal: To electronically document patient history for a new Pain Management Service patient in the PMIDS database.

Overview: The use case begins when the provider creates a record for a newly admitted PMIDS patient. The provider enters patient-specific historical information, including demographics, diagnoses, and surgeries, in the data entry form of the PMIDS database. Upon verification of accuracy, the provider indicates that the data should be saved in the PMIDS database. If a record has already been created for the patient in the PMIDS database, the provider will initiate the Query Data Use Case. The Use Case ends when the provider indicates a desire to exit the Use Case OR when there are no more new patients to be entered into the PMIDS database.

Priority (user): High

Rank (analyst): High

Preconditions:
1. Patient admitted to the Pain Management Service.
2. Patient has been assigned an account number.
3. Patient history, including demographics, diagnoses, and surgeries, is available to the provider from the patient, patient's family, and/or paper medical record.

Actor Action	System Responsibility
Provider chooses Enter Data in PDA	System displays a blank data entry form with the appropriate fields for a newly admitted patient.
Provider enters name and medical record number of newly admitted patient into data entry form.	System displays name and medical record number of newly admitted patient in appropriate fields.
Provider enters patient history, including demographics, diagnoses, and surgeries into data entry form.	All newly entered patient historical data is displayed.in appropriate fields
Provider verifies accuracy of entered data.	System displays entered data.
Provider chooses Save Data function at APN workstation.	All newly entered data is stored in the PDA on a patient-specific basis.

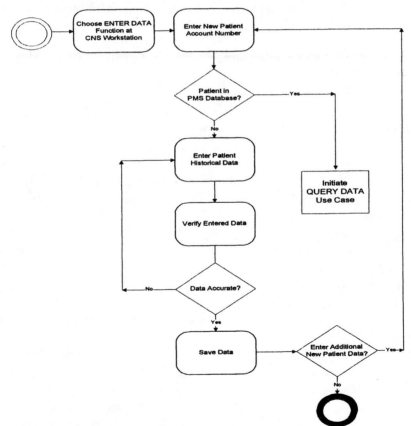

FIGURE 7.10 Activity Diagram.

4. A Microsoft Access database, *(http://www.microsoft.com)*, with the appropriate fields, has been created.
5. The provider is authorized to access the PMIDS system.

Postconditions:
1. Patients admitted to the Pain Management Service have historical data, including demographics, diagnoses, and surgeries, accurately entered into the database.
2. Patients will be identified in the PMIDS database by name and medical record number.

Use Case Summary:

Each use case is diagrammed, described, pathways developed, and activity diagrams drawn to reflect the user's needs. The process is considered "complete" when *the product of value* for the *user* is clear to both developers and users on the project team. For the "enter data" use case, the products of value are reflected in the postconditions above, or those things that should result when the use case is completed. In the example provided, the products of value include specific kinds of data for patients on the Pain Management Service, and an ability to find their records by name and/or medical record number in the PMIDS database. This seems fundamental to any good documentation system but is not always known by technical developers. Even this level of requirements documentation needs further detail in order to develop a usable system, and functional specifications take the process to the next level of detail.

EXAMPLE VIRTUAL TEAM PROJECT: FUNCTIONAL REQUIREMENTS AND CONCEPT DIAGRAM

Functional Requirements *(Selected Section of a Pain Management Documentation Application)*

(Credit and thanks to Kevin Sprecher, Kathy Samon, MJ Petersen—class of 1999)

Functional specifications act as a blueprint for software program development, and provide a description of the purpose of the software. Specifications may or may not include user interface screens and implementation details, depending on the application and the project team's skills in developing those details. The example below is part of the user interface description for a pain management documentation "parent form." The parent form acts as the reference point for the multiple assessments and interventions that are documented on multiple subforms.

In this PDA application, for every patient encounter, one parent form is created. Subsequent assessments and interventions are given a unique subform. For a thorough description of the elements that are being documented, however, a class diagram is needed.

Concept (class) Diagram

A class or concept diagram describes the manner in which the concepts interact with each other. These diagrams include the relationships of the objects within the system. The attributes of the classes are presented in this diagram also. The diagram below demonstrates the concept/class diagram for the parent form for the Pain Management Team's documentation. For the arrows shown, the number one (1) indicates that there is one patient for any number (indicated by *) of therapies, interventions, assessments, etc.

Historically, a large gap existed between technical developers and clinical experts. Clinical knowledge is complicated, frequently nonstandardized, and dynamic; clinical knowledge evolves quickly with changes in clinical research and therapeutic insights. Technical developers cannot be expected to know or learn this clinical knowledge, nor should the clinician be expected to learn the technical details of the systems they utilize for patient care. It is also true that technical knowledge is complicated, frequently nonstandardized and always dealing with dynamic "moving target" new hardware. What must be learned, is a standard communication process for technology-intensive information systems being developed for clinicians. The modeling of use cases, functional specifications, activity, and class/concept diagrams allow for the clinician to more easily communicate system requirements to technical developers. The important translation role that helps clinical and technical experts better communicate is central to many nursing informatics positions. A more productive and efficient development process is enhanced when the informatics nurse specialist is able to model the desired system with clinical users input, and then translate those models and requirements when meeting with technical experts.

```
┌─────────────────────────────────────┐
│                                     │
│        Patient Intervention Subform │
│                                     │
│  Field (field type)                 │
│  1.  Patient Medical Record (History) Number │
│       (freeform text)               │
│  2.  Patient Last Name (freeform text) │
│  3.  Intervention #1 (lookup list - see right) │
│  4.  Intervention #1 Date/Time (date/time field) │
│  5.  Intervention #1 notes (freeform text) │
│  6.  Intervention #2 (lookup list - see right) │
│  7.  Intervention #2 Date/Time (date/time field) │
│  8.  Intervention #2 notes (freeform text) │
│  9.  Intervention #3 (lookup list - see right) │
│  10. Intervention #3 Date/Time (date/time field) │
│  11. Intervention #3 notes (freeform text) │
│                                     │
└─────────────────────────────────────┘
```

Version Note: The intervention subform now allows for up to three interventions with one access of the subform. The previous version only allowed one

Intervention Lookup List
Explanation/Discussion
Demonstration
Handout given
Reinforcement
Music Therapy
Massage Therapy
Relaxation Technique
Imagery
Bolus Fentanyl
Bolus Lidocaine
Stop infusion
Hold infusion
Hang new solution
Changed tubing
Increased infusion/dose
Decreased infusion/dose
Called for pump delivery
Called for pump pickup
Added adjunct therapy
Changed catheter hub
Changed catheter filter

FIGURE 7.11 Functional Requirements.

Project Learning Value (This is an excerpt from student evaluations)

The project was large enough to encompass all phases of project management, although on a small scale. Iterative development was fruitful in producing improvement at every step of the analysis, development, implementation, and evaluation. The project was an excellent opportunity to examine one possible use of hand-held technology in the delivery of patient care. The entire project was of value for all of the team members, relative to their own experience level. Specific learning experiences included:

- Working through all phases of systems life cycle
- Collaboration with advanced practice nurses, in two separate locations, involved in the treatment of cardiac patients
- Development of data entry forms for data collection via handheld technology
  1. Defining current processes and information collected

2. Designing forms to facilitate data collection by use of selection lists when standardized data choices existed
3. Development of advanced database skills

- Learning from iterations and feedback from end users.

Team Process

Challenges for a team working on a project of this nature included leadership, individual work pace, rhythm, and communication. These might be problematic for many teams, but were part of the success of this team because:

- The leadership role freely moved within the team, depending on the activity focus and individual strengths.
- The work pace and rhythm of team members seemed to mesh and complement each other.
- Constructive confrontation and conflict resolution skills were improved over the course of two semesters.
- Communication was easy, direct, and constructive, resulting in improvements in all phases and deliverables throughout the entire project.

PLANNING FOR THE FUTURE

In the Information Age, value is placed on the individual who can creatively acquire and manage information. Innovation is crucial for survival, and imitation is a sure recipe for disaster. Thus any curriculum that does not teach students how to synthesize and creatively apply material is an antique. Putting lecture notes on-line and then giving multiple choice tests on-line must not be the new model of nursing informatics education. The "tell them and test them" model of education, in which students are viewed as empty vessels waiting to be filled with knowledge from the "Sage on the Stage," is a relic from the period when the value of creative thinking was less important than filling classroom and teaching rosters.

Despite the availability and relatively low cost of technology, most schools are behind the times in thinking about genuinely new course designs, collaborative learning experiments, and a major overhaul of the roles of professor and student. The question for nursing informatics

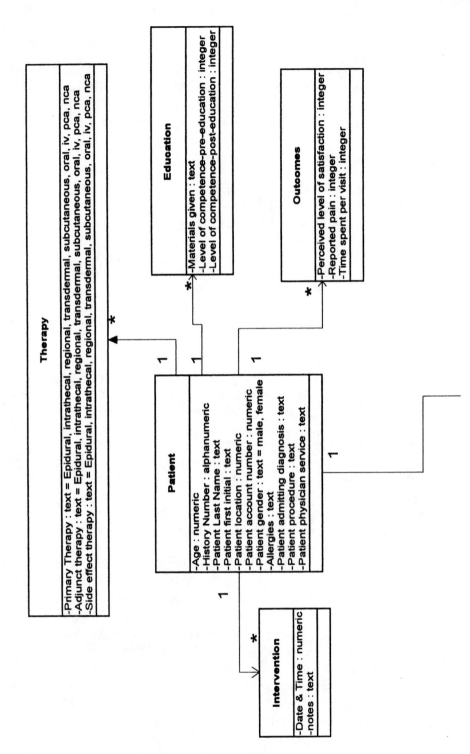

FIGURE 7.12 Class Diagram/Concept Model.

Assessment

*

- Reported pain : numeric
- systolic blood pressure : numeric
- diastolic blood pressure : numeric
- Activity : text = resting, coughing, turning, ambulating/wallking, nothing
- Heart Rate : numeric
- Level of consciousness : text = agitated, alert-cooperative, confused, unconscious
- Respiratory rate : numeric
- Learning readiness : text = receptive/unreceptive
- Learning barriers : text = cognitive, emotional, physical, language, none
- Constipation : text = yes/no
- Headache : text = yes/no
- Pruritis-local : text = yes/no
- Pruritis-general : text = yes/no
- Nausea : text = yes/no
- Vomiting : text = yes/no
- Backache at site : text = yes/no
- Anticoagulation : text = none, Heparin SC, Heparin infusion, Lovenox, Coumadin, Warfarin, Dextran
- sensory band begin : text
- sensory band end : text
- bromage scale : numeric
- Catheter aspiration : text = N/A, negative, positive, positive with heme, positive with glucose, positive with heme and glucose

education is quite clear: Do colleges and universities facilitate learning and advance knowledge OR provide courses that are simply filled with students to generate credit hour revenues? The very survival of our profession may depend on the answer.

While it is difficult to plan and design programs based on new paradigms and technology, there are some basic principles that can be followed as we move forward through the discovery process. Values that facilitate a new pedagogy include humility, intellectual honesty, openness, receptiveness to new ideas, treating others with dignity and respect, and recognizing and using everyone's unique knowledge and abilities. These values lead to two basic principles for adult education (Brockett & Heimstra, 1994):

1. It is important to empower adults to take personal responsibility for their own learning
2. Instructional activities should be based on learners' perceived needs.

From these two principles, Duke's program strives to be a pioneering effort that guides the development of nursing informatics courses where learning is focused on practical problem solving. Nurses' previous problem solving and clinical experience is an invaluable resource for future learning in informatics. As we recognize nurse learners enter an informatics (and any other) teaching/learning setting with a wide range of skills, abilities, and attitudes, we will begin to consider each student's unique contribution in the instructional planning process. Additionally, while the traditional semester *does* constrain learning opportunities, the learning environment should attempt to allow each student to learn at a pace best suited to the individual. With increasing flexibility in the learning place, it is important to help students continuously assess their progress and make feedback an inherent part of the learning process.

Duke's Nursing Informatics students have completed their program from all corners of the continent, including Canada and Alaska. Most of Duke's alumni work in Nursing Informatics positions within health care (primarily hospital settings), but others work for vendors and consulting firms. Just a few of the many roles they now play in nursing informatics include:

- Work with various standards groups to represent nursings' needs
- Analysis and requirements documentation for user needs
- Nurse end-user advocates and user support—liaison between clinical and technical personnel
- Translation and/or development of HL7 interfaces
- Full systems life cycle support management (supervising their departments)
- Configuring/building a variety of applications using vendor-based clinical systems
- Enterprise wide strategic planning for new system(s) selection
- Project management leadership for multiple enterprise-wide systems projects
- Consulting for multiple clients with regard to clinical systems and applications issues

In an era of chaos and controversy with regard to health care services, computerized patient records, and emerging patient privacy legislation at the federal level, highly qualified and competent informatics nurse specialists are needed in a variety of roles within the health care system. Duke University School of Nursing's Informatics program will continue to strive to meet new millennium challenges that result in innovative pedagogy and improved problem solving for nursings' future.

REFERENCES

Adams, D. (1979). *The hitchhiker's guide to the galaxy.* New York: Random House, Wings Books.

American Nurses Association [ANA] (1994). *The scope of practice for nursing informatics.* Washington, DC: American Nurses Publishing.

American Nurses Association [ANA] (1995). *Standards of practice for nursing informatics.* Washington, DC: American Nurses Publishing.

Booch, G., Jacobsen, I., & Rumbaugh, J. (1999). *The unified modeling language user guide.* Menlo Park, CA: Addison-Wesley Publishers.

Brownstein, B. (1998). *Discovering a new pedagogy for a new medium.* [On-Line] Available: *http://home.ubalt.edu/bbrownstein/papers/webteaching.html.*

Brockett, R. G., & Hiemstra, R. (1994). *Self-direction in adult learning:*

Perspectives on theory, research, and practice. London and New York: Routledge.

Davidson, J. D., & Rees-Mogg, W. (1997). *The sovereign individual: How to survive and thrive during the collapse of the welfare state.* New York: Simon & Schuster.

Hiemstra, R., & Sisco, B. (1990). *Individualizing instruction: Making learning personal, empowering, and successful.* San Francisco: Jossey-Bass.

Markee, N. P. P. (1996). *Managing curricular innovation.* New York: Cambridge University Press.

8

Post-Master's Education:
A Model for a Nursing
Informatics Fellowship
Rita D. Zielstorff

For many years, nurses who worked with information systems "learned by doing." With no formal education programs available in nursing informatics, nurses adapted the skills and knowledge they already had with respect to project management, change management, and interpersonal relations. They learned about information systems technology from technical colleagues, or took courses in business schools in computer programming or systems analysis. They occasionally had peer support from colleagues in other agencies. In the 1980s, a few books on computers in nursing appeared, but experience was the main teacher.

Today, the nurse who wants to make a career in informatics has many choices for obtaining the necessary knowledge and skills; several of these choices are described in this book. One frequently chosen route is to obtain a Master's Degree in Nursing Informatics, or a Master's Degree in Nursing with a concentration in informatics. Some nurses choose this route having already worked in an information systems position, wanting a deeper knowledge of informatics-related topics as they relate to nursing. These nurses emerge from their academic program with both the knowledge and skills to perform at a high level of competency.

The nurse who has no experience in informatics prior to entering a Master's program emerges with good exposure to the *knowledge* in the field. However, academic programs can provide only limited experience for skills such as analyzing user needs, diagramming information flow, determining and documenting functional requirements, designing data bases, using project management software, designing the user interface, training users, evaluating system impact, and many others that are the substance of the practice of informatics. An extra year in which to practice these skills in a real-world environment where mentoring and support are provided could help the nurse to launch his or her informatics career on solid footing. This paper describes the author's experience with conducting a series of one-year, post-Master's Nursing Informatics Fellowships at two separate institutions.

DEVELOPMENT OF THE PROGRAM

The Post-Master's Nursing Informatics Fellowship program at Partners HealthCare System originated at the Massachusetts General Hospital (MGH) in 1993. The Information Systems Department of the Department of Nursing had the responsibility to implement and support automated information systems for nursing, such as systems for patient classification and nurse scheduling. The nurses in this department had varied educational backgrounds, but none had any course work in nursing informatics. All, however, were quite experienced at system selection, user training, system implementation, and system support

The hospital had earlier contracted with an information systems vendor to codevelop a total automated system with an emphasis on providing clinical decision support using relatively structured clinical data. As plans for the rollout proceeded, nursing leadership discussed what skills nurses at all levels would need in order to take advantage of the technology. It became clear that knowledge about nursing informatics principles would be essential, at least among those nurses who would be working most closely with codeveloping the system. The director of nurses and the author conceived the idea of a 1-year post-Master's Fellowship in Nursing Informatics that would have mutual benefits for both MGH and the Fellow. The Fellow would be expected to bring and share the latest knowledge about nursing informatics, while our staff would assist the new informatics graduate in gaining skills needed in practice. Consultation with recruiters, employers, faculty at Master's programs, and new graduates themselves confirmed that such a program would increase the value of the participant to potential employers. None of those consulted knew of such a program in this country. The National Library of Medicine sponsors a program of pre- and post-doctoral traineeships in medical informatics with an emphasis in research through institutional grants, and an individual traineeship in applied informatics, (*http://www.nlm.nih.gov/pubs/factsheets/trainedu. html*, Sept. 1999). However, we could find no description at that time of a hospital-based post-Master's program in nursing informatics with an emphasis on skill building.

A proposal was developed and approved by the MGH Nursing Executive Committee to offer a 1-year Post-Master's Fellowship in Nursing Informatics, with the position supported by special funds. Leadership of the program was assigned to the author. The purposes of the program were to

1. foster the development of Informatics Nurse Specialists who are well-grounded in both the theory and practice of the application of computers to nursing;
2. foster the exchange of information and knowledge regarding nursing informatics; and
3. promote the Massachusetts General Hospital as a center for the practice of nursing informatics.

The proposed program had these characteristics:

- The Fellow would be paid an annual stipend with full employee benefits, with the understanding that the Fellowship period would be for 1 year only. The amount of the stipend was competitive with post-doctoral fellowships in other nursing and health-related areas.
- The Fellow would have the opportunity to explore current activities at the hospital, and in particular in the Department of Nursing, related to data, decision support, and automated systems.
- The director of the MGH/Harvard Medical School Laboratory of Computer Science (LCS), in which the author was also employed, offered its facilities as a laboratory. The Fellow could explore projects in the LCS if desired, and participate in grant proposal preparation and grant reporting to the extent that those activities were currently taking place.

- After the exploratory period, the Fellow would be expected to develop specific goals for self-development that would be reviewed with the program director on a quarterly basis, and revised as appropriate.
- The Fellow would be expected to choose one or two projects on which to focus, and to play a role that would serve both his or her own needs for development as well as the needs of the hospital.
- The Fellow would be expected to lead a weekly seminar for nurses in the information systems department on current trends and issues in nursing informatics.
- The Fellow would be expected to co-tutor a semester-long survey course in nursing informatics to be given at the MGH Institute of Health Professions. The Fellow would also be provided with opportunities to give talks and guest lectures at local meetings and at local universities.

With the position approved and the program broadly outlined, it was time to begin soliciting applicants. A special relationship was formed with faculty and leaders at the University of Maryland School of Nursing, which had a thriving Master's program in Nursing Informatics. Impending graduates of the Master's program were informed about the Fellowship and its application requirements. By December 1992, the first fellow, Margaret (Mimi) Hassett, was selected. In February 1993, she was welcomed at MGH with much enthusiasm at a formal tea given in her honor.

EARLY EXPERIENCE WITH THE PROGRAM

A true risk taker, Ms. Hassett realized that she would be helping us to mold the program, and had faith that she would learn something useful along the way. One of her goals was to gain experience with grant-funded research projects, so her first activity was to prepare a grant request for the NLM Fellowship in Applied Informatics. Another goal was to learn more about the ethical impacts of informatics in health care, so she joined the MGH's multidisciplinary Ethics Core Interest Group. Her goal to gain more experience with papers and presentations was realized by giving a number of presentations at venues such as Regis College in Boston, University of

Massachusetts (Worcester), Bellarmine College in Louisville, and several at MGH. She prepared and published a manuscript describing the fellowship program in Medsurg Nurse (Hassett, 1994). She gained experience in project management by leading the planning of a day-long continuing education program in nursing informatics. She developed skills in analysis of nursing information system requirements by preparing a proposal to extend the patient classification system to the emergency department. She participated in a software selection project to choose a bibliographic management program for LCS. She learned the principles of graphical user interface design through her participation in a grant-funded project to provide access to guidelines knowledge related to pressure ulcers. She became an acknowledged resource for connecting with the outside electronic world by sharing her skills with using the Internet and other electronic communication methods.

After acquainting herself with the projects underway in the Department of Nursing and at LCS, she chose to focus on two: the Nursing Minimum Data Set Database Project and the Problem-Based Access to Guidelines Knowledge project. The former was a project to abstract medical record data of a randomly selected group of patients to look for the presence of the items included in the Nursing Minimum Data Set (Werley, Lang, & Westlake, 1986). The latter was a grant-funded project to structure data from text guidelines in order to provide quick answers to clinicians at the point of care about patient-specific problems (Zielstorff, Barnett, Fitzmaurice, Estey, Hamilton, 1996).

During the final quarter of her fellowship, preparation began for separation from the program. Ms. Hassett was encouraged to formalize her career goals, target desired positions, and prepare her resumé. We forwarded known position openings to her, provided recruiters' names, practiced interviewing skills with her, and of course, supplied a recommendation. Ms. Hassett gave a positive review of her experience, and at the end of it, took a position at St. Elizabeth's Medical Center as Senior Systems Analyst, ultimately becoming Nursing MIS Coordinator there.

At MGH, review of the experiences of the prior year showed that the major purposes of having a hospital-based fellowship program could be achieved. Rather than draining hospital resources, the Fellow can extend them. Nurses at the hospital gained exposure to trends and issues in nursing informatics, and skills in using Internet resources for information gathering and communication. The projects that the Fellow worked on benefited from her participation, and indeed, some would not have been achieved at all without her leadership. The Nursing Executive Committee gave permission to search for ways of funding the program on a permanent basis.

EVOLUTION OF THE PROGRAM

While the hospital development office searched for ways of funding the program permanently, special funds were used to support a second 1-year fellowship. A second University of Maryland graduate, Emily Welebob, was accepted into the program. Ms. Welebob's goals and interests were supported through working on projects such as conducting a study of clinicians' use of a paperless obstetrics record (Welebob, Zielstorff, Chueh, & Barnett, 1996), implementing an experimental system for point-of-care decision support for pressure ulcers (Zielstorff, Barnett, et al., 1996), conducting a review of vendors for a provider order-entry system, and implementing and evaluating an automated resource for patient instructions (Welebob & Tronni, 1996). In addition, she played a key role in supporting an analysis of problem terms from three nursing classification systems (Zielstorff, Tronni, Basque, Griffin, & Welebob, 1998). Sharing an office with a member of the hospital's nursing information systems staff encouraged informal exchange of information and skills.

Once again, review of the year's experience showed that the 1-year fellowship program could augment the novice informatician's skills while contributing meaningfully to the hospital's information systems agenda. At the end of her program, Ms. Welebob took a position as a consultant with First Consulting Group.

TRANSITION TO PARTNERS HEALTHCARE SYSTEM

When the author left Massachusetts General to join the parent corporation, Partners HealthCare System, the Nursing Informatics Fellowship Program was instituted as a permanently funded position in the Clinical Information Systems Research and Development group in Partners Information Systems. Now, yearly soliciting of candidates would no longer be dependent on finding funds for the position. The mission, purpose, and loose structure of the fellowship remained similar, but the range of mentors and experiences broadened to include all Partners entities, including acute care, home-based, and ambulatory care practices.

Successive Fellows Andrew Awoniyi, R.N., N.D., Beth Tomasek, R.N., M.S., and Cheryl Reilly, R.N., Ph.D., brought diverse backgrounds, talents, goals and achievements to the program. Some of their accomplishments are cited in Awoniyi (1997), Awoniyi, Zielstorff, Teich, & Goldszer (1997), Tomasek, Sagoo, & Xiao (1998), Tomasek (1998), Reilly (1999), and Reilly, Zielstorff, Fox, O'Connell, Carroll, et al. (in press). Though each candidate's experience was unique in terms of learning achieved, projects supported, and post-fellowship employment, the program continued to be positively evaluated by fellows themselves, their preceptors, and the program's organizers.

WHAT MAKES A GOOD FELLOW?

The number of candidates applying for the fellowship increased yearly. This forced us to formalize our selection process, and to provide documentation to support our selection of one candidate over another. Each candidate who expressed an interest in the program was asked to supply the following:

- A letter of application which includes the applicant's reason for interest in the program and career objectives. (We want to be sure that the candidate intends to pursue a career in nursing informatics.)
- A current CV or resumé
- A transcript of completed graduate courses
- A list of courses that remain to be completed before graduation
- Written recommendations from the school's Program Director, from a Faculty member, and from a preceptor of a practicuum or field experience.

From these materials, we learned whether the candidates are able to express their goals clearly, and whether the goals are in line with what we could provide. We also could see whether they did well in school, what kind of experience they had before going into the

Master's program, and whether their teachers and preceptors believed they would succeed in the fellowship.

We required a structured personal interview, whether conducted by telephone or face to face. Over the years, we have learned what characteristics bode well for a productive fellowship, so we structured the interview to see whether the candidate appeared to have the following skills and abilities:

- Ability to work both independently and as a team member, with strong interpersonal skills
- Ability to set learning goals, identify opportunities for learning, and monitor progress toward goals
- Ability to integrate into a large organization, and form relationships conducive to carrying out change
- Ability to organize and manage multiple tasks, with appropriate priority-setting
- Demonstrated proficiency in word processing; beginner skills in database management, project management and spreadsheet software
- Beginner skills in at least one high-level programming language
- Familiarity with research methods, with beginner skills in data synthesis and presentation
- Strong analytical and problem-solving skills, with skills in using tools such as flowcharting to help define problems
- Good writing skills; beginner verbal presentation skills
- Flexibility to adapt to changing demands, ability to change focus, manage transitions

While not all successful candidates have all of these skills to the same degree, we believed that the candidate who is deficient in several of the areas mentioned above would require more help and support than we were able to give. This will undoubtedly lead to an unsatisfactory experience for the fellow and a frustrating experience for us.

TRANSITION TO THE VENDOR ENVIRONMENT

The author has left Partners HealthCare System and joined an internet healthcare company. A Nursing Informatics Fellowship Program is being designed. The vendor environment will provide a different experience from that of an academic medical center, yet the overall goal remains: to provide the novice informatics practitioner with an experience that augments needed skills while supporting the goals of the sponsoring organization. We fully expect that, as in the prior programs, we will provide fellows with diverse projects and experiences, gently support their learning, and proudly follow their post-fellowship achievements.

REFERENCES

Awoniyi, A. (1997). *Assessing the supplemental information needs of nurses —A replicative study.* Poster session presented at Rutgers College of Nursing Fifteenth Annual International Nursing Computer and Technology Conference, Atlantic City, NJ.

Awoniyi, A., Zielstorff, R. D., Teich, J. M., & Goldszer, R. C. (1997). *Assessment of information activities of physicians utilizing an electronic patient record.* Unpublished manuscript.

Hassett, M. (1994). Nursing informatics fellowship. *MEDSURG Nursing, 3*(1), 73–74.

Reilly, C. A. (1999). Examining the symptom experience of hospitalized patients using a pen-based computer. *Proceedings AMIA '99 Annual Symposium,* 364.

Tomasek, B. A. (1998). Evaluation of vendor-supplied product for patient instructions. Unpublished report.

Tomasek, B. A., Sagoo, N., & Xiao, Y. (1998). Telemedicine: Pilot evaluation of user satisfaction survey tool. In C. G. Chute (Ed.), *Proceedings AMIA '98 Annual Symposium,* 1085.

Welebob, E., & Tronni, C. (1996). End-user satisfaction of a patient education tool: Manual vs computer generated tool. *Computers in Nursing, 14*(4), 235–238.

Welebob, E., Zielstorff, R. D., Chueh, H., & Barnett, G. O. (1996). *Provider-patient interactions during obstetrical clinical encounters utilizing a desktop clinical workstation.* Unpublished manuscript.

Werley, H. H., Lang, N. M., & Westlake, S. K. (1986). Nursing minimum data set conference: executive summary. *Journal of Professional Nursing, 2*(4), 217–224.

Zielstorff, R. D., Barnett, G. O., Fitzmaurice, J. B., Estey, G., Hamilton, G., Vickery, A., Welebob, E., & Shahzad, C. (1996). A decision support system for prevention and treatment of pressure ulcers based on AHCPR guidelines. In J. J. Cimino, (Ed.), *Proceedings 1996 AMIA Annual Fall Symposium,* 562–566.

Reilly, C. A., Zielstorff, R. D., Fox, R. L., O'Connell, E. M., Carroll, D. L., Conley, K. A., Fitzgerald, P., Kahleret Eng, T., martin, A., Zidik, C. M., & Segal, M. (accepted for publication). A knowledge-based patient assessment system: conceptual and technical design. Accepted for publication in *Proceedings 2000 AMIA Annual Fall Symposium.*

Zielstorff, R. D., Tronni, C., Basque, J, Griffin, L. R., & Welebob, E. M. (1998). Mapping nursing diagnosis nomenclatures for coordinated care. *Image: Journal of Nursing Scholarship, 30*(4), 369–373.

9

Standards for Electronic Health Records and Clinical Decision Support Systems
Suzanne Bakken

Standards are a vital component of the development and implementation of electronic health records and clinical decision support systems. Without standards it is not possible to represent, exchange, manage, or integrate health care data, information, and knowledge among disparate computer-based systems for the delivery, management, and evaluation of health care. One would certainly find little disagreement with a statement that characterized the current information system environment in the United States today as one of disparate computer-based systems! Additionally, although the activities aimed at improving health care processes and outcomes have changed through the years (e.g., quality improvement, quality management, process re-engineering, evidence-based practice), the need for data interchange and data integration has remained central.

Standards are at the core of interoperability, which is "the ability of two or more systems or components to exchange information and to use the information that has been exchanged" (Institute of Electrical and Electronics Engineers, 1990). Interoperability can be further differentiated into functional interoperability, that is, the ability to exchange information, and semantic interoperability, that is, the ability to use exchanged information (Beeler, 1999a). Because of the significance of enabling standards for electronic health records and clinical decision support (application areas that are frequently the focus of nursing informatics practice), knowledge and skills in health care standards are a core competency for nursing informatics.

Standards-related content and opportunity for application of knowledge and skills should be incorporated into nursing informatics curricula.

What are the types of standards that are needed for interoperability? The International Standards Organization (ISO) Open Systems Interconnection (OSI) communication architecture specifies the need for standards representing seven layers of connectivity, ranging from the physical connection (Level 1) to the application level (Level 7) (Rose, 1989). Although standards related to all seven layers of connectivity are essential, the specific purposes of this chapter are to provide a broad overview of application level standards that enable electronic health records and clinical decision support systems and to describe implications for nursing informatics education.

Following a brief introduction to standards organizations and standards development processes, four specific categories of standards will be reviewed. These are standards related to:

1. health care terminologies;
2. transmission of messages;
3. decision support rules; and
4. privacy, confidentiality, and security.

Because standards are evolving rapidly, the focus will be on guiding principles and sources of standards rather than on detailed descriptions of specific standards. Lastly, suggestions for content and methods of incorporating standards content into nursing informatics curricula will be given.

STANDARDS DEVELOPMENT ORGANIZATIONS AND STANDARDS DEVELOPMENT PROCESSES

Although standards development activities related to electronic interchange of health care data and information have spanned decades, the complexity of the current health care environment and subsequent value of information for the delivery, management, and evaluation of health care has increased the interest in and demand for standards. In recent years, efforts have been further fueled by the mandate for standards in the Health Insurance Portability and Accountability Act (HIPAA) of 1996 (Department of Health and

Human Services. Office of the Assistant Secretary for Planning and Evaluation. Administrative simplification, 1996). Table 9.1 lists selected organizations engaged in the standards development or facilitation process and designates which categories of standards within the purview of this chapter are addressed by the organization. Organizations such as Health Level 7 (HL7), American Society for Testing and Materials (ASTM), and the International Standards Organization (ISO) have a broad range of standards-related activities. Other groups have focused their efforts on standards that are particularly relevant to the purpose of the organization (e.g., American Nurses Association [ANA] and Computer-based Patient Record Institute [CPRI]).

Hammond and Cimino (2000) delineate four ways that a standard can be produced. In the ad hoc method, interested stakeholders develop and mutually agree upon a standard specification, for example, the American College of Radiology/National Electrical Manufacturers Association (ACR/NEMA) DICOM standard (Bidgood, & Horii, 1992). In contrast, the de facto method occurs when a single vendor controls enough market share to make its product the standard, for example, Microsoft Windows. The Minimum Data Set for Long-Term Care required by the Health Care Financing Administration represents the government-mandate method (HCFA, 1997). The predominant method for the creation of health care standards is the consensus method. HL7 and Accredited Standards Committee (ASC) X12 exemplify this approach.

Standards-related testimonials presented before groups such as the American National Standards Institute-Health Informatics Standards Board (ANSI-HISB) and the National Council for Vital and Health Statistics (NCVHS) suggest that the recent progress towards interoperability is significant.

HEALTH CARE STANDARDS

Standardized Health Care Terminologies

Standardized health care terminologies (i.e., the set of terms representing a system of concepts (International Standards Organization, 1990)) are necessary to reliably and validly describe, support, and analyze health care processes and outcomes. During the last several decades, extensive development of standardized health care and

TABLE 9.1 Organizations Focused on Standards Development or Facilitation

Organization	1	2	3	4
Accredited Standards Committee (ASC) X12 and X12N	✓	✓		
American College of Radiology/National Electrical Manufacturers Association (ACR/NEMA)	✓	✓		
American Dental Association (ADA)	✓			
American Medical Association (AMA)	✓			
American Nurses Association (ANA)	✓			
American National Standards Institute Health Care Informatics Standards Board (ANSI-HISB)	✓	✓	✓	✓
American Society for Testing and Materials (ASTM)	✓	✓	✓	✓
College of American Pathologists/SNOMED	✓	✓	✓	✓
Computer-based Patient Record Institute (CPRI)	✓			✓
European Standardization Committee (CEN)	✓	✓	✓	✓
Health Care Financing Administration (HCFA)	✓	✓	✓	✓
Health Level 7 (HL7)	✓	✓	✓	✓
Institute of Electrical and Electronic Engineers (IEEE)			✓	✓
International Standards Organization (ISO)	✓	✓	✓	✓

1 = Standardized Health Care Terminologies, 2 = Decision Support, 3 = Messaging, 4 = Privacy, Confidentiality, and Security

nursing terminologies has occurred. (American Medical Association, 1993; Brown, O'Neil, & Price, 1998; Grobe, 1996; International Council of Nurses, 1999; Johnson & Maas, 1997; Kleinbeck, 1996; Martin & Scheet, 1992; McCloskey & Bulechek, 1996; NANDA, 1994; Ozbolt, 1996; Saba, 1992; Spackman, Campbell, & Cote, 1997; Werley & Lang, 1988) Table 9.2 summarizes the content of selected terminologies related to aspects of the nursing process. The significance of these developments is epitomized in the following statement from Norma Lang: "If you cannot name it, you cannot control it, finance it, teach it, research it, or put it into public policy" (Clark & Lang, 1992, p. 109).

Given the obvious need for the information and the availability of multiple terminologies, one might ask, "Why are standardized terminologies not universally implemented in computer-based systems?" A number of organizations and terminology experts have proposed criteria or standards related to the suitability of terminologies for incorporation into computer-based systems (Table 9.3). Evaluation studies of standardized terminologies against these criteria provide some answers to this question.

The evaluation criteria can be broadly conceptualized into two categories. The first category comprises criteria that focus on the content of a terminology in relationship to the needs of a particular domain (e.g., breadth of coverage, abstract vs. atomic terms) (American Nurses Association, 1999; Chute, Cohn, & Campbell, 1998). In contrast, the second set of criteria focuses on the computability (e.g., concept-orientation, non-ambiguous representation, support for synonymy) and evolution (e.g., concept permanence, non-semantic identifiers) of a terminology over time (CEN ENV 12264, 1995; Chute et al., 1998; Cimino, 1998).

The primary focus of nursing terminology development has appropriately been on the collection and categorization of nursing concepts. Evaluations of terminologies against domain coverage criteria support several conclusions:

- Standardized nursing terminologies demonstrate broad coverage for nursing diagnoses, nursing interventions, and nursing-sensitive outcomes. (Henry, Warren, Lange, & Button, 1998)
- Terminologies not specifically designed for nursing include some terms used by nurses to document problems (e.g., SNOMED International) and interventions (e.g., Physician's Current Procedural Terminology Codes) (Griffith & Robinson, 1992; Henry, Holzemer, Randell, Hsieh, & Miller, 1997; Henry, Holzemer, Reilly, & Campbell, 1994; Lange, 1996).
- In addition to the abstract terms (e.g., nursing diagnoses and nursing interventions) predominant in nursing classification systems, less abstract, that is, more atomic, terms (e.g.,

TABLE 9.2 Standardized Terminologies for Representing Concepts Relevant to the Nursing Domain

Terminology	Assess	Diagnose	Intervene	Outcome[1]
Nursing				
Home Health Care Classification (Saba, 1992)[2]	✓	✓	✓	✓
International Classification of Nursing Practice (International Council of Nurses, 1999)		✓	✓	✓
NANDA Taxonomy 1 (NANDA, 1994)[2]		✓		
Nursing Intervention Lexicon And Taxonomy (Grobe, 1996)			✓	
Nursing Interventions Classification (McCloskey & Bulechek, 1996)[2]			✓	
Nursing Outcomes Classification (Johnson & Maas, 1997)[2]				✓
Nursing Minimum Data Set (Werley & Lang, 1988)[2]		✓	✓	✓
Omaha System (Martin & Scheet, 1992)[2]	✓	✓	✓	✓
Patient Care Data Set (Ozbolt, 1996)[2]		✓	✓	✓
Perioperative Data Set (AORN, 1997)[2]		✓	✓	✓
Health care				
International Classification of Diseases (1992)	✓	✓		
National Health Service Clinical Terms (Brown, O'Neil, & Price, 1998)	✓	✓	✓	✓
Physicians' Current Procedural Terminology (American Medical Association, 1993)			✓	
SNOMED RT (Spackman, Campbell, & Cote, 1997)[2]	✓	✓	✓	✓

[1] Includes goal setting and/or outcome evaluation; [2] Recognized by American Nurses Association

TABLE 9.3 Sources for Criteria Addressing Suitability of Terminologies for Implementation in Computer-Based Systems

- American National Standards Institute—Health Information Standards Board (Chute, Cohn, & Campbell, 1998)
- American Nurses Association (American Nurses Association, 1999)
- American Society for Testing and Materials (ASTM E1284-96, 1996)
- Computer-Based Patient Record Institute (Chute et al., 1998)
- Desiderata for Controlled Medical Vocabulary (Cimino, 1998)
- European Committee for Standardization (CEN ENV 12264, 1995)
- Health Level 7 (*http://www.hl7.org*)
- International Standards Organization (International Standards Organization, 1990

symptoms and specific nursing activities) are also needed to represent nursing concepts (Campbell, Carpenter, Sneiderman, et al., 1997; Henry, Holzemer, Reilly, et al., 1994; Henry & Mead, 1997).

The findings of these evaluation studies document that the existing set of standardized terminologies provides terms for the majority of concepts required to represent nursing domain content in computer-based systems. Additionally, recent efforts have focused on the development of terminologies that include atomic terms for nursing concepts (e.g., Patient Care Data Set (Ozbolt, 1996), International Classification of Nursing Practice (International Council of Nurses, 1999), SNOMED RT (Spackman et al., 1997)).

Standardized nursing terminologies, and in fact, health care terminologies with few exceptions (e.g., SNOMED RT and Logical Observation Identifiers, Names, and Codes [LOINC] (Huff, Rocha, McDonald, et al., 1998)), have not been developed with the second category of criteria in mind, but primarily for other purposes (e.g., classification) (Henry & Mead, 1997). A useful discrimination among terminologies by purpose is provided by Spackman et al. (1997) who contend that some terminologies are optimized for ease of use (i.e., interface terminology, e.g., locally developed terms for order sets), whereas others are optimized for statistical classification (i.e., administrative terminology, e.g., Physician's Current Procedural Terminology (American Medical Association, 1993)) or nonambiguous concept representation and facilitation of computer-based terminology management and data re-use (i.e., reference terminology, e.g., SNOMED RT). Standardized nursing terminologies frequently serve as both interface and administrative terminologies.

Because they have not been developed to function as a reference terminology, standardized nursing terminologies do not meet the criteria (e.g., non-ambiguous concept representation, concept permanence) that primarily relate to such a terminology. In recognition of the need for a reference terminology that would complement existing standardized nursing terminologies and facilitate integration and aggregation of data represented in different terminologies, recent efforts have focused on incorporating nursing concepts into SNOMED RT and developing structures to support a reference terminology for nursing (Hardiker & Rector, 1998; Bakken, Cashen, & O'Brien, 1999; Warren, Mead, Button, Androwich, & Henry, 1999).

Standardized terminologies meeting the criteria related to suitability for implementation into computer-based systems are essential to achieve the goal of semantic interoperability for electronic health records and clinical decision support systems. Recent efforts towards consensus and collaboration around standardized terminologies suggest that terminologies are evolving, and that with a substantial commitment of resources the goal of semantic interoperability is attainable for at least subsets of data in the near future.

Decision Support

In addition to standardized terminologies for representing health care concepts, standards are required to represent knowledge bases that generate common decision support functions such as alerts, interpretations, screens, etc. The Arden Syntax for medical logic systems is the focus of this brief overview. An outcome of a 1989 retreat of medical informatics groups held to examine issues about knowledge base sharing, the syntax was later adopted by ASTM (Hripcsak, 1994a). Activities related to Arden have recently been incorporated into HL7 (HL7 Clinical Decision Support and Arden Syntax Technical Committee, 1998) and in 1999, the Arden Syntax was designated as an ANSI-accredited standard.

To date, the scope of the Arden Syntax has been limited to knowledge bases that can be represented as a set of discrete modules (Hripcsak, 1994a). Each Medical Logic Module (MLM) contains sufficient information to make a single decision. Types of knowledge that can be represented in an MLM include:

1. contraindication alerts (e.g., allergic to sulfa);
2. client management suggestions (e.g., increase potassium supplement if on digoxin and serum potassium is low);
3. data interpretations (calculate fractional excretion of sodium);
4. treatment and research screening protocols (e.g., meets inclusion criteria for clinical trial); and
5. diagnosis scores (e.g., at risk for fall).

Each MLM comprises three major categories of slots: maintenance, library, and knowledge (Hripcsak, 1994b). As shown in Figure 9.1, the maintenance category includes identifying information about the MLM (e.g. title, institution, Arden Syntax version). The purpose of the MLM and its related citations (an optional slot) are contained in the library component of the MLM. The core of the MLM is the knowledge representation that consists of four major functional components:

1. evoking event (i.e., trigger);
2. logic or algorithm;
3. action; and
4. data mapping.

The Penicillin Alert MLM illustrated in Figure 9.1 is triggered when an order is written for a penicillin medication. The logic executed in this simple alert is focused on the determination of whether or not a penicillin allergy is present. If it is true that a penicillin allergy exists, then an action is triggered. Depending upon the level of urgency associated with the action, a message may appear immediately on the provider's computer screen (e.g., contraindicated drug, drug-drug interaction) or be sent via e-mail (e.g., a message to the clinical trial study coordinator that a patient meets the eligibility screening for a research study). Data mapping is illustrated by the relationship between the text contained within the curly braces, for

MLM Template   MLM for a Penicillin Allergy Alert
maintenance:
    title: _____;; (some brief description)
    mlmname:_____;; (a unique name for the MLM)
    arden:_____;; (Version of Arden)
    version:_____;; (MLM version; always start with 1.00)
    institution: _____;; (institution name)
    author: _____;; (author name)
    specialist: ;; (always blank to start)
    date: _____;; (date of creation or revision)
    validation: testing;; (always start with testing)
library:
    purpose: (why would the MLM be used)
    _____.;;

    explanation: (how does the MLM work)

    _____
    _____.;;
    keywords:_____;; (words or phrases that describe the MLM)
    citations: ;; (optional list of citations related to MLM)
knowledge:
    type: data-driven;; (always data-driven)
    data: (define the event used in the evoke spot and read data for the logic spot)
    /* _____*/ (comment)
    _____; (data mapping)
    /* _____*/ (comment)
    _____;
    ;;
    evoke:
    _____;; (what event should trigger the MLM)
    logic: (create the logic necessary to carry out the task and conclude true
      when you want to write a message)

    _____
    _____;
    ;;
    action: (write a message, combining narrative text and calculated values)
    _____;
    urgency: ———;; (designate the urgency of the message where 1 is low and
    99 is high)
end:

FIGURE 9.1 Medical Logic Module (MLM) example.

The left side of the figure shows the slots of a MLM and describes their purposes. The right side illustrates an instantiation of the slots for a penicillin allergy alert.

maintenance:
    title: Check for penicillin allergy;;
    mlmname: pen_allergy;;
    arden: ASTM-E1460-1995;;
    version: 1.00;;
    institution: Columbia-Presbyterian Medical Center;;
    author: George Hripcsak, M.D.;;
    specialist: ;;
    date: 1991-03-18;;
    validation: testing;;
library:
    purpose:
        when a penicillin is prescribed, check for an allergy.;;
    explanation:
        This MLM is evoked when a penicillin medication is ordered. An alert is
        generated because the patient has an allergy to penicillin recorded.;;
    keywords: penicillin; allergy;;
    citations: ;;
knowledge:
    type: data-driven;;
    data:
        /* an order for a penicillin evokes this MLM */
        penicillin_order := event {medication_order where class = penicillin};
        /* find allergies */
        penicillin_allergy := read last {allergy where agent_class = penicillin};
    ;;
    evoke:
        penicillin_order;;
    logic:
        if exist(penicillin_allergy) then
                conclude true;
        endif;
        ;;
    action:
        write "Caution, the patient has the following allergy to penicillin docu-
mented:
    urgency: 50;;
end:

This figure was adapted with permission from Hripcsak, G. (1994b). Writing
Arden Syntax Medical Logic Modules. *Computers in Biology and Medicine,*
24(5), 331–363.

example, {medication_order where class=penicillin}, which represents the institution-specific terms, and the MLM terms (i.e. penicillin_order).

Demonstrations support the usefulness of the Arden Syntax for MLMs as a standard for sharing discrete knowledge bases. Development of MLMs centered on nursing concepts is needed to provide decision support for phenomena that are primarily the concern of nursing, for example, management of urinary incontinence, pressure ulcer risk screening, falls prevention.

Transmission of Messages

Central to the functionality for electronic health records and clinical decision support systems envisioned in the 1991 Institute of Medicine report (Dick & Steen, 1991), is a set of standards related to the syntax and semantics of messages exchanged among systems. As noted in Table 9.1, several organizations have developed messaging standards. In this chapter, the HL7 Message Development Framework (MDF) for Version 3 of the HL7 Standard is used as an exemplar of messaging standards development.

The MDF methodology is based upon object-oriented analytical processes and employs standardized notation (i.e., Unified Modeling Language [UML] (Fowler, 1997)) supported by a standard modeling tool, Rational Rose. The relationships among models in the MDF are shown in Figure 9.2 (Beeler, 1999b).

Requirements analysis is focused on the intended use of the standard and is represented as a Use Case Model. This is complemented by a domain analysis represented as an information model. There are several levels of information models involved. The Reference Information Model (RIM) is a coherent, shared information model that is the source for the data content for all HL7 messages. The HL7 RIM has been developed through a consensus process including harmonization activities aimed at incorporating the work of domain subject groups (e.g., Long-term care/Home care, Orders/Observations) into the RIM. Work groups focused on a particular domain (e.g., Patient Care, Blood Bank) develop messages for that domain and work with a subset of relevant concepts which is represented as a Domain Information Model (DIM).

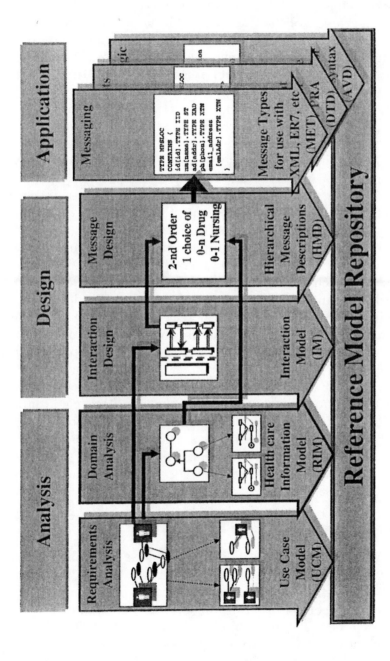

FIGURE 9.2 *Relationships among the models in the HL7 message definition framework.*
Reprinted with permission from Beeler, G. W. (1999b). Taking HL7 to the next level. *MD Computing, 16(2)*, 21–24.

The requirements and domain analyses are followed by the design phase. The design of the Interaction Model specifies definition of information flows and communication roles of system components. The design of a message includes the creation of a Message Information Model (MIM) which is a subset of the DIM, the development of a Message Object Diagram (MOD), and the specification of a Hierarchical Message Definition (HMD). As compared to earlier versions of HL7, the MDF is aimed at producing messages that support semantic interoperability at the level of the terminology. Thus, the role of standardized terminologies in "naming" the concepts in the messages is crucial. Towards this objective, liaisons from the HL7 Vocabulary Technical Committee work with each domain group (e.g., Patient Care) to assist with terminology-related issues and to assure that terminologies being considered to represent the concepts meet the HL7 criteria for compliant vocabularies.

The Implementation Technology Specification (ITS) describes the manner in which HL7 messages are sent using a particular implementation technology (Klein, 1999). These specifications include: 1) methods of encoding the messages; 2) rules for the establishment of connections and transmission timing; and 3) procedures for dealing with errors. The ITS may also include a specified application programming interface. The HL7 Version 3 implementation technology will initially be Extensible Markup Language (XML).

The tremendous commitment from stakeholders (e.g., vendors, users, professional organizations, consultants, government, etc.) towards HL7 messaging standards is evidenced by the widespread adoption of earlier versions of the standard and by productivity of the organization as it applies the MDF to message development and related activities.

Privacy, Confidentiality, and Security

The ability to systematically link from disparate computer-based systems, data and information related to a particular individual or group of individuals, affords new opportunities to improve health care, but also raises concerns regarding the confidentiality and security of health care data and information (Etzioni, 1999). As a basis for understanding the issues surrounding policy adoption and standards development, a number of groups and organizations have proposed definitions for the central concepts.

The following definitions are used for this chapter:

Privacy—the right of individuals to keep information about themselves from being disclosed to anyone (CPRI Work Group on Confidentiality, 1995b).

Confidentiality—the act of limiting disclosure of private matters; maintaining the trust that an individual has placed in one which has been entrusted with private matters (CPRI Work Group on Confidentiality, 1995a).

Security—the means to control access and protect information from accidental or intentional disclosure to unauthorized persons and from alteration, destruction, or loss (CPRI Work Group on Confidentiality, 1995a). Aspects of security have been more explicitly differentiated in an Institute of Medicine (Donaldson & Lohr, 1994) report as:

> *Data/information security*—the result of effective protection measures that safeguard data/information from undesired occurrences and exposure to accidental or intentional disclosure to unauthorized persons, accidental or malicious alteration, unauthorized copying, loss by theft and/or destruction by hardware failures, software deficiencies, operating mistakes, or physical damage by fire, water, smoke, excessive temperature, electrical failure, or sabotage.

> *System security*—the result of all safeguards including hardware, software, personnel policies, information practice policies, disaster preparedness, and oversight of these components.

The importance of this area of standards development is reflected not only by the attention and scrutiny of the American public, but in the multiple and diverse groups drafting guiding principles or standards. The IEEE-USA Medical Technology Policy Committee published a comparison of principles across 10 sources and proposed 28 draft principles on privacy, confidentiality, and security (Buckovich, Rippen, & Rozen, 1999). Their analysis revealed 11 principles that were consistent across the majority of sources. As shown in Table 9.4, areas of agreement include those principles focused on individual rights and on the need for policies, procedures, and regulations as well as for education regarding the aforementioned.

On the other hand, one of the most contentious areas related to privacy, security, and confidentiality is the scientific and public debate surrounding the need for and nature of a universal identifier for health care to facilitate access to and linkage of health care information. A universal health care identifier (UHID) is "a means to provide positive recognition of a particular individual for all people in a population. A universal health care or patient identifier provides the identifier for use in health care transactions (ASTM Committee E-31 on Computerized Systems. Subcomittee E31.12 on Medical Records, 1995)." ASTM E1714-95 specifies the desired properties of a UHID (ASTM, 1999). A federally sponsored comparison of the extent to which a variety of identifier schemes (not necessarily UHIDs), such as biometrics (e.g., retinal scanning), probabilistic matching, and approaches based upon the social security number, included the properties, suggested that a security-enhanced number based upon the social security number met the majority of the criteria. Opponents of this approach cite a concern that health care data will potentially be linked with financial records (Etzioni, 1999) or argue that sophisticated informatics approaches are superior to a simple identifier (Szolovits & Kohane, 1994).

Technology offers excellent methods for tasks such as:

1. linking personally identifiable or dis-identified health information;
2. restricting access:
3. encrypting data;
4. authenticating users;
5. digital signatures; and
6. maintaining audit trails.

However, experts agree that technology is only part of the solution to issues of privacy, confidentiality, and security (Computer Science and Telecommunication Board, 1997; CPRI Work Group on Confidentiality, 1995b; Donaldson & Lohr, 1994). This is reflected in the principles in Table 9.4. Need for institutional change at the federal policy level and in organizations is emphasized by Etzioni (1999) who states "often the most effective way to treat an ethical or sociopo-

TABLE 9.4 Consistent Principles Across Sources Related to Privacy, Confidentiality, and Security

- Individuals have a right to the privacy and confidentiality of their health information.
- Outside the doctor-patient relationship, health information that makes a person identifiable shall not be disclosed without prior patient informed consent or authorization. Nine entities have exceptions to this principle, for allowing disclosure without prior informed consent or authorization, including emergencies, current legal and public health requirements, law enforcement, and research.
- All entities with exposure or access to individual health information shall have security/privacy/confidentiality policies, procedures, and regulations (including sanctions) in place that support adherence to these principles.
- Individuals have a right to access in a timely manner their health information. Three entities have exceptions to the right to access, for special state law requirements or for the protection of the individual.
- Individuals have a right to control the access and disclosure of their health information and to specify limitation on period of time and purpose of use.
- Employers have a right to collect and maintain health information about employees allowable or otherwise deemed necessary to comply with state and federal statutes (e.g., ERISA, drug testing, worker's compensation). However, employers shall not use this information for job or other employee benefit discrimination.
- All entities involved with health care information have a responsibility to educate themselves, their staff, and consumers on issues related to these principles (e.g., consumers' privacy rights).
- Individuals have a right to amend and/or correct their health information. One entity has an exception and refers to the exception as under certain circumstances.
- Health information and/or medical records that make a person identifiable shall be maintained and transmitted in a secure environment.
- An audit trail shall exist for medical records and be available to patients on request. Five entities support an audit trail but do not specifically mention that patients shall have access to it.
- Support for these principles needs to be at the federal level.

Adapted with permission from Buckovich, S. A., Rippen, H. E., & Rozen, M. J. (1999). Driving toward guiding principles: A goal for privacy, confidentiality, and security of health information. *Journal of the American Medical Informatics Association, 6*(2), 122–133.

litical problem is to modify or recast institutions, rather than to rely solely or even chiefly upon the aggregation of millions of actions by newly informed individuals" (p. 20).

IMPLICATIONS FOR NURSING INFORMATICS CURRICULA

Because of the foundational role of health care standards to the development and implementation of electronic health records and clinical decision support systems, a nursing informatics curriculum must include content related to standards. An example of the integration of standards content into courses in a nursing informatics educational program is shown in Table 9.5. Learning activities from those courses that are specific to the four categories of standards discussed in this chapter are listed in Table 9.6.

Beyond those areas of content listed in the example, knowledge and skills in structured markup languages, particularly XML, and the creation of document type definitions (DTDs) would also be useful for some aspects of standards work. In addition, didactic content should be complemented by focused "real-world" opportunities (e.g., externships, practica) for application of standards-related knowledge and skills.

SUMMARY

In recent years, there has been significant progress towards the development of standards that enable electronic health records and clinical decision support systems. In order to facilitate the adoption of relevant standards, knowledge and skills in the area of standards must be a core competency of clinical nursing informatics practice. In addition, it is vital that nurses with appropriate knowledge and skills participate in the standards development process so that the standards adequately support nursing domain content. Without the exchange and use of nursing data among computer-based systems (i.e., semantic interoperability), it will be impossible to support the delivery of nursing care and to determine the contributions of nursing to health care processes and outcomes.

TABLE 9.5 Integration of Standards Content into a Nursing Informatics Curriculum[1]

Course	Standards topics covered
Introduction to health care informatics	• Standards development organizations and processes
	• Introduction to standardized health care terminologies
	• Privacy, confidentiality, and security
Decision making and decision support systems	• Arden Syntax for medical logic modules
Abstraction and modeling	• Use case models
	• Information models
	• Interaction models
	• Unified modeling language
Health care concept representation	• Standardized health care terminologies
	• Terminology models
	• Formal approaches to concept representation (e.g., conceptual graphs)
Consumer health informatics	• Privacy, confidentiality, and security

[1] School of Nursing, University of California, San Francisco

TABLE 9.6 Sample Assignments Related to Standards[1]

Standardized health care terminologies
- Match terms documented in chart with standardized health care terminologies using the Unified Medical Language System (UMLS) Metathesaurus (oral presentation)
- Critique an existing standardized health care terminology using CPRI/ANSI-HISB criteria and Cimino's Desiderata (oral presentation)
- Propose a terminology model for a set of health care concepts based upon their defining characteristics and represent them using conceptual graph grammar (paper)
- Model a selected set of health care concepts using a distributed computer-based modeling and conflict resolution environment (laboratory exercise)

Decision support
- Develop a rule for a nursing decision support system and represent it using Arden syntax (section of oral presentation and paper related to design of a decision support system)

Messaging
- Create a use case model, information model, and interaction model for a health care process that requires communication among computer-based systems (small group work over the duration of a quarter-long course with successive oral presentations)

Privacy, confidentiality, and security
- Compare and contrast two approaches (e.g., biometrics and probabilistic matching) for linking health care information (paper)
- Critique a security education program or policy from a clinical institution (paper)

[1]School of Nursing, University of California, San Francisco

REFERENCES

American Medical Association (1993). *Physician's current procedural terminology.* Chicago: Author.

American Nurses Association (1999). *Recognition criteria for data sets, classification systems, and nomenclatures.* Washington DC: American Nurses Association.

ASTM Committee E-31 on Computerized Systems. Subcomittee E31.12 on Medical Records (1995). *ASTM E1714 Guide for the properties of a universal health identifier.* West Conshohocken, PA: American Society for Testing and Materials.

ASTM *E1714-95 (1999). Standard guide for properties of a universal healthcare identifier.* West Conshohocken, PA: American Society for Testing and Materials.

ASTM E1284-96 (1996). *Guideline for construction of a clinical nomenclature for the support of electronic health records.* West Conshohocken, PA: American Society for Testing and Materials.

Bakken, S. B., Cashen, M. S., & O'Brien, A. (1999). Evaluation of a type definition for representing nursing activities within a concept-oriented terminologic system. In N. Lorenzi (Ed.), *Proceedings of the 1999 AMIA Annual Symposium. Journal of the American Medical Informatics Association Symposium Supplement.* Philadelphia, PA: Hanley & Belfus, Inc.

Beeler, G. W. (1999a). *Presentation to the National Committee on Vital and Health Statistics.* Available: *http://www.hl7.org* [1999, July].

Beeler, G. W. (1999b). Taking HL7 to the next level. *MD Computing, 16*(2), 21–24.

Bidgood, W. D. J., & Horii, S. C. (1992). Introduction to the ACR-NEMA DICOM Standard. *Radiographics, 12,* 345–355.

Brown, P. J. B., O'Neil, M., & Price, C. (1998). Semantic definitions of disorders in Version 3 of the Read Codes. *Methods of Infomation in Medicine, 37*(4–5), 415–419.

Buckovich, S. A., Rippen, H. E., & Rozen, M. J. (1999). Driving toward guiding principles: A goal for privacy, confidentiality, and security of health information. *Journal of the American Medical Informatics Association, 6*(2), 122–133.

Campbell, J., Carpenter, P., Sneiderman, C., Cohn, S., Chute, C., & Warren, J. (1997). Phase II evaluation of clinical coding schemes: Completeness, taxonomy, mapping, definitions, and clarity. *Journal of the American Medical Informatics Association, 4*(3), 238–251.

CEN ENV 12264 (1995). *Medical informatics—Categorial structure of systems of concepts—Model for representation of semantics.* Brussels: CEN.

Chute, C. G., Cohn, S. P., & Campbell, J. R. (1998). A framework for comprehensive terminology systems in the United States: Development guidelines, criteria for selection, and public policy implications. ANSI Healthcare Informatics Standards Board Vocabulary Working Group and the Computer-based Patient Records Institute Working Group on Codes and Structures. *Journal of the American Medical Informatics Association, 5*(6), 503–510.

Cimino, J. J. (1998). Desiderata for controlled medical vocabularies in the twenty-first century. *Methods of Information in Medicine, 37*(4–5), 394–403.

Clark, J., & Lang, N. M. (1992). Nursing's next advance: An international classification for nursing practice. *International Nursing Review, 39,* 109–112.

Computer Science and Telecommunication Board (1997). *For the record: Protecting electronic health information.* Washington, DC: National Academy Press.

CPRI Work Group on Confidentiality, P., & Security (1995a). *Guidelines for establishing information security education policies at organizations using computer-based records.* Schaumburg, IL: Computer-based Patient Record Institute.

CPRI Work Group on Confidentiality, P., Rivacy & Security (1995b). *Guidelines for information security education programs using computer-based patient records.* Schaumburg, IL: Computer-based Patient Record Institute.

Department of Health and Human Services. Office of the Assistant Secretary for Planning and Evaluation. Administrative simplification (1996). *ASPE Web site.* Available: *http://aspe.os.hhs.gov/admnsimp* [1999].

Dick, R. S., & Steen, E. B. (Eds.) (1991). *The computer-based patient record: An essential technology for health care.* Washington, D.C.: National Academy Press.

Donaldson, M. D., & Lohr, K. N. (Eds.) (1994). *Health data in the information age: Use, disclosure, and privacy.* Washington, DC: National Academy Press.

Etzioni, A. (1999). Medical records: Enhancing privacy, preserving the common good. *Hastings Center Report, 29*(2), 14–23.

Fowler, M. (1997). *UML distilled: Applying the standard object modeling language.* Reading, MA: Addison-Wesley.

Griffith, H. M., & Robinson, K. R. (1992). Survey of the degree to which critical care nurses are performing Current Procedural Terminology-coded services. *American Journal of Critical Care, 1,* 91–98.

Grobe, S. J. (1996). The Nursing Intervention Lexicon and Taxonomy: Implications for representing nursing care data in automated records. *Holistic Nursing Practice, 11*(1), 48–63.

Hammond, W. E., & Cimino, J. J. (2000). Standards in medical informatics. In E. H. Shortliffe & L. Perreault (Eds.), *Medical informatics: Computer applications in medical care and biomedicine.* New York: Springer-Verlag.

Hardiker, N. R., & Rector, A. L. (1998). Modeling nursing terminology using the GRAIL representation language. *Journal of the American Medical Informatics Association, 5*(1), 120–128.

HCFA (1997). Medicare and Medicaid; resident assessment in long term care facilities—HCFA. Final rule. *Federal Register, 62*(246), 67174–67213.

Henry, S. B., Holzemer, W. L., Randell, C., Hsieh, S. F., & Miller, T. J. (1997). Comparison of nursing interventions classification and current procedural terminology codes for categorizing nursing activities. *Image, 29,* 133–138.

Henry, S. B., Holzemer, W. L., Reilly, C. A., & Campbell, K. E. (1994). Terms used by nurses to describe patient problems: Can SNOMED III represent nursing concepts in the patient record? *Journal of the American Medical Informatics Association, 1,* 61–74.

Henry, S. B., & Mead, C. N. (1997). Nursing classification systems: Necessary but not sufficient for representing "what nurses do" for inclusion in computer-based patient record systems. *Journal of the American Medical Informatics Association, 4*(3), 222–232.

Henry, S. B., Warren, J., Lange, L., & Button, P. (1998). A review of the major nursing vocabularies and the extent to which they meet the characteristics required for implementation in computer-based systems. *Journal of the American Medical Informatics Association, 5*(4), 321–328.

HL7 Clinical Decision Support and Arden Syntax Technical Committee (1998). *Arden Syntax for Medical Logic Systems.* [On-Line] Available: *http://www.hl7.org* [1999, 7/27/99].

Hripcsak, G. (1994a). The Arden Syntax for Medical Logic Modules: Introduction. *Computers in Biology and Medicine, 24*(5), 329–330.

Hripcsak, G. (1994b). Writing Arden Syntax Medical Logic Modules. *Computers in Biology and Medicine, 24*(5), 331–363.

Huff, S. M., Rocha, R. A., McDonald, C. J., De Moor, G. J. E., Fiers, T., Bidgood, W. D., Jr., Forrey, A. W., Francis, W. G., Tracy, W. R., Leavelle, D., Stalling, F., Griffin, B., Maloney, P., Leland, D., Charles, L., Hutchins, K., & Baeziger, J. (1998). Development of the LOINC (Logical Observation Identifier Names and Codes) Vocabulary. *Journal of Medical Informatics Association, 5*(3), 276–292.

Institute of Electrical and Electronics Engineers (1990). *IEEE Standard Computer Dictionary: A compilation of IEEE standard computer glossaries.* New York, NY.

International Council of Nurses (1999). *ICNP Update.* Geneva, Switzerland: International Council of Nurses.

International Standards Organization (1990). *International Standard ISO 1087: Terminology—Vocabulary.* Geneva, Switzerland: International Standards Organization.

Johnson, M., & Maas, M. (Eds.) (1997). *Nursing Outcomes Classification (NOC).* St. Louis: C.V. Mosby.

Klein, W. T. (1999). *Introduction to HL7 Version 3.* Tutorial presented at the Health Level 7 Winter Working Group Meeting, Orlando, FL.

Kleinbeck, S. V. M. (1996). In search of perioperative nursing data elements. *AORN Journal, 63*(5), 926–931.

Lange, L. (1996). Representation of everyday clinical nursing language in UMLS and SNOMED. In J. J. Cimino (Ed.), *Proceedings of the 1996 AMIA Fall Symposium (Formerly SCAMC). Journal of the American Medical Informatics Association Symposium Supplement* (140–144). Philadelphia, PA: Hanley & Belfus, Inc.

Martin, K. S., & Scheet, N. J. (1992). *The Omaha System: Applications for Community Health Nursing.* Philadelphia: WB Saunders.

McCloskey, J. C., & Bulechek, G. M. (1996). *Nursing Interventions Classification* (2nd ed.). St. Louis: C. V. Mosby.

NANDA (1994). *Nursing diagnoses: Definitions & classification 1995–1996.* Philadelphia, PA: North American Nursing Diagnosis Association.

Ozbolt, J. G. (1996). From minimum data to maximum impact: Using clinical data to strengthen patient care. *Advanced Practice Nursing Quarterly, 1*(4), 62–69.

Rose, M. T. (1989). *The open book, a practical perspective on OSI.* Upper Saddle River, NJ: Prentice-Hall.

Saba, V. K. (1992). The classification of home health care nursing: Diagnoses and interventions. *Caring Magazine, 11*(3), 50–56.

Spackman, K. A., Campbell, K. E., & Cote, R. A. (1997). SNOMED RT: A Reference Terminology for Health Care. In D. R. Masys (Ed.), *Proceedings of the 1997 AMIA Annual Symposium, Journal of the American Medical Informatics Association, Symposium Supplement* (pp. 640–644). Philadelphia: Hanley & Belfus, Inc.

Szolovits, P., & Kohane, I. (1994). Against simple universal health-care identifiers. *Journal of the American Medical Informatics Association, 1*(4), 316–319.

Warren, J. J., Mead, C. N., Button, P., Androwich, I., & Henry, S. B. (1999). Development and evaluation of the Loose Canon Model of nursing interventions using Unified Modeling Language. In N. Lorenzi (Ed.), *Proceedings of the 1999 AMIA Annual Symposium, Journal of the American Medical Informatics Association, Symposium Supplement.* Philadelphia: Hanley & Belfus, Inc.

Werley, H. H., & Lang, N. M. (Eds.) (1988). *Identification of the Nursing Minimum Data Set.* New York: Springer.

10

The Learning Circle:
A Collaborative Model to Promote
Nursing Informatics Education
Diane Skiba

The evolution of nursing informatics education has emulated the development of information systems in health care. In nursing, computer education introduced in the 1970s focused on computer basics and applications related to the automation in health care. In the 1980s, computer education evolved into what is now known as nursing informatics education. This evolution transformed the focus away from computer literacy and the automation process focus to an emphasis on informatting nursing, that is making nursing visible through the integration of computer, information and nursing sciences. This chapter will trace the development of an international informatics model within the historical context of nursing informatics education. The international model demonstrates the collaboration between two schools, University of Colorado Health Sciences Center School of Nursing (UCHSC-SON) and Hogeschool Holland, to foster the development of nursing informatics education. This chapter describes three distinct phases of development over an 8-year time span. The chapter concludes with four guiding principles for the development of collaborative international models for nursing informatics education.

HISTORICAL CONTEXT

The history of nursing informatics education is less than 25 years old with the first course offered in 1976 at State University of New York at Buffalo. This undergraduate elective course created by Dr. Judith

Ronald emphasized computer fundamentals, basics of systems analysis and design, and a review of applications in health care (Ronald, 1979). This course served as a foundation for the development of numerous courses across the globe. The National League for Nursing facilitated this development by publishing two monographs. The first monograph provided guidelines for basic computer education in nursing (Ronald & Skiba, 1987). The second monograph was a series of papers that addressed recommended informatics competencies for nurses (Peterson & Gerdin-Jerlag, 1988). During this period, courses focused primarily on three main components: computer basics, applications in nursing education, administration, practice, and research; and interactive hands-on experiences with commonly available software packages such as databases, spreadsheets, and word processing. Courses were available throughout the United States (State University of New York, Boston University, Georgetown University, Case Western Reserve, University of Texas at Austin, University of California at San Francisco).

Towards the end of 1980s, computer education for nurses evolved into the now current informatics education. The work of Graves and Corcoran (1989) and the creation of graduate programs specializing in nursing informatics at the University of Maryland and University of Utah served as a catalyst to reshape and define nursing informatics education. Nursing informatics education moved beyond computer literacy and applications focus to a discipline that combined principles from computer and information sciences to support the informatting of nursing. This evolution reflected a similar trend in the development of information systems in health care. Applications were evolving from automation of data to applications that manipulated and transformed data into meaningful information. Curriculum models (Romano & Heller, 1988) helped to shape the next generation of informatics courses. Aarts (1989) reported one of the first post-graduate nursing informatics program in the Netherlands. Courses began to appear internationally in Australia, New Zealand, and throughout Europe in the early 1990s.

The introduction of the ANA Scope of Practice and Standards in Nursing Informatics Practice hastened the development of informatics courses but there remained only three formal informatics programs (University of Maryland, University of Utah, Case Western Reserve). Two additional programs targeted toward nurse educators facilitated the growth of nursing informatics education during the 1990s. The first was the HBO Nurse Scholars Program started in 1990. The short-term goal of the HBO Nurse Scholars program was to facilitate the integration of informatics into the curriculum (Skiba, Simpson, & Ronald, 1992). The long-term goal was to establish a means for future generations to be educated in the use, design, implementation and management of information systems in the clinical arena (Skiba, Simpson, & Roland, 1992). The other program was the European Nursing Informatics Summer School started in 1991. This intensive week-long summer school allowed nurses to work in small teams with the support of a Tutor and Co-Tutor. For the first 4 years of the program, teams were divided across topics in nursing education, practice, and administration. The nursing education team focused on the development of a nursing curriculum in informatics. In the last decade, the European Nursing Informatics Summer School graduates and developers were responsible for the continued growth of this discipline throughout Europe. Many participants have created courses (Chambers, 1994; Saranto, 1998) and both tutors and participants have been involved in the Nightingale Project (Mantas & Dounavis, 1997). The Nightingale project, started in 1996, created an implementation plan for training the nursing profession in using and applying health care information systems. It is the repository of nursing informatics knowledge across Europe (*http://www. dn.uoa.gr/nightingale*).

This brief history of nursing informatics education provides the framework for the development on an international model of informatics education. This idea for this model germinated in 1992 and has evolved to an institutional partnership between the UCHSC-School of Nursing and the Hogeschool Holland. What follows is a description of this evolution across three distinct phases over the last 8 years.

PHASE I: HUMBLE BEGINNING (1992–1993)

The collaboration between the Hogeschool Holland and the University of Colorado Health Sciences Center School of Nursing began with a sharing of ideas between two colleagues (Skiba & Springer, 1995). This dialogue began at the Second European Nursing Informatics Summer School in Stirling, Scotland. The dialogue shared ideas about content, curriculum, and teaching methods. The exchange allowed each person to describe their educational programs and to place these programs within the context of nursing education within each of the respective countries. Here are the initial descriptions of the schools during this first phase.

The Hogeschool Holland is a polytechnic school located in a place called Diemen near Amsterdam. The bachelor program for nursing had three major fields of study: nursing, nursing administration and nursing informatics. The bachelors program for nursing informatics was a 3-year part-time program designed to allow a working nurse to take classes one day a week. The program prepared nursing informatics specialists for one of three major roles: analyst, innovator and advisor, or educator. This means that a nursing informatics specialist, in the view of the Hogeschool Holland, must have knowledge about nursing, nursing theories, organisational science, project management, economics, didactics (teaching), and communication skills (Skiba & Springer, 1995). In addition, the nursing informatics specialist must have sufficient knowledge about information science and informatics so he/she can be involved in building information systems and can be an advocate for nursing.

The School of Nursing at the University of Colorado Health Sciences Center offers the B.S., M.S., joint M.S./M.B.A., and Ph.D. degrees as well as the Doctor of Nursing (N.D.) program. The Baccalaureate program was designed to prepare students for entry into the nursing profession in generalist practice. The N.D. was an advanced generalist professional nursing degree for non-nursing college graduates. The Master's program prepared nurses for advanced practice in areas of specialty such as adult-health, community health, nursing administration, midwifery, psychiatric-mental health, and primary health care. The Ph.D. program was designed to prepare nurse scholars who are highly motivated toward advancing the art, science and practice of the nursing discipline.

This exchange, maintained by e-mail over the next year, was solidified at the Third European Nursing Informatics Summer School in Genk, Belgium. At this point, course outlines were shared along with learning activities and textbooks. The sharing of information necessitated the translation of Dutch materials into the English language. It was clear at this meeting that the next step was to explore opportunities for our students to dialogue with each other about the nature of nursing informatics in both countries. To facilitate this dialogue, the students accessed an electronic bulletin board system operated by the UCHSC School of Nursing. The electronic bulletin board system (Denver Free-Net) was used as an educational support for both on-campus and distance learners. It was also used as an alternative method for the delivery of health care to consumers in the state of Colorado (Skiba & Mirque, 1994). The system allowed registered users to read text-based information, retrieve and download text-based files, search databases, and use various communication mechanisms such as e-mail, chat functions (two or three users can simultaneously chat on the system), discussion groups, and computer conferencing. This electronic bulletin board predated the World Wide Web and served as a mechanism for the students in Holland to communicate with the students in Colorado. The goals of these initial student interactions were twofold: to assess if students could communicate with relative ease and to identify any infrastructure needs before learning assignments were required in existing courses.

PHASE II: (1994–1997) STUDENT GLOBAL COLLABORATIVE LEARNING PROJECT

The success of the student interactions in the initial phase provided a fruitful environment for the development of a pilot project. The pilot would provide collaborative learning experiences for students enrolled in the Hogeschool Holland Nursing Informatics Program and those students enrolled in one of two electives courses offered at the UCHSC School of Nursing. Another key ingredient was the availability of a computer conferencing system that both schools could access through the Internet. The Denver Free-Net provided e-mail and computer conferencing for both schools. The faculty had a face-to-face meeting after the recent Nursing Informatics '94 International Symposium and generated the following mission and goals of the Global Collaborative Learning Project (Skiba & Springer, 1995). The mission of this project was threefold. First, this project would foster collaborative learning experiences for nursing students across two schools of nursing. Second, the project would facilitate the exchange of nursing knowledge across countries. Lastly, the project would strengthen nursing's role in the development of the global information infrastructure. To achieve this mission, several goals were proposed. The goals were:

1. to establish the technical requirements for collaborative distance learning;
2. to foster communication among faculty and students across schools of nursing;
3. to encourage the exchange of nursing knowledge via collaborative assignments;
4. to facilitate the development of nursing informatics curriculum; and
5. to provide a foundation for future nursing exchange programs.

Since the UCHSC School of Nursing only offered two electives in nursing informatics, the decision was made to use the overview course on nursing informatics for the pilot project. This course provided an overview of nursing informatics and included such topics as: information science basics, clinical information systems, community health management information systems, health-oriented telecommunications, management systems, multimedia/instructional technologies, legal and ethical issues, and nursing informatics roles. Computer conferencing, in-class seminars, and hands-on computer experiences were the instructional techniques used throughout this course. Approximately one-third of the classes were conducted via computer conferencing so the students could asynchronously work on learning assignments over the Internet.

Each semester (fall and spring) that the overview course was offered, the two groups of students would work together on a series of joint learning activities. These learning activities included such assignments as the development of criteria to assess web-based health education programs for consumers, an exchange of informatics roles and availability of positions in each country, a review of telehealth applications in each respective country, and the creation of pertinent web sites for nursing informatics. Course evaluations continually highlighted the positive strengths of these collaborative learning efforts. As time passed, access to the Internet and ease of use with electronic communications greatly facilitated class assignments.

PHASE III: INSTITUTIONAL PARTNERSHIP (1998–PRESENT)

The continued success of these pilot projects and numerous changes in the two institutions precipitated the next phase of this international model. First, both institutions experienced changes in leadership and in the organizational structures of the schools of nursing. For the Hogeschool Holland, the major change was progression from a polytechnic institution to a university for higher education. The University was now organized into different working units and with an updates educational mission. The University had some 9,000 registered students in more than 50 different degree programs. The Hogeschool Holland is a publicly funded University and is recognized by the Dutch Ministry of Education. It has four basic principles for sound education: identity, innovation, internationalization, and informatics. The school stresses the following principles:

1. to do justice to people from numerous culture and denominations
2. to coordinate its courses to actual practice
3. to respond to the growing demand for internationally prepared professionals
4. to prepare students for a future in which knowledge of computerization is indispensable.

The University of Colorado Health Sciences Center School of Nursing, under new leadership, celebrated its 100th year anniversary in 1998. The School of Nursing continued to offer all four-degree programs but significantly revised the curricula across these four programs. Four significant changes had the most effect on the collaborative efforts between the schools. First, the leadership strongly believed this collaboration needed to move from individual efforts to an institutional partnership between the two schools. To this end, a memorandum of agreement was signed. Second, the nursing curricula across all four programs incorporated a new focus called the human technology interface. This new focus expanded the school's view of technology beyond information technologies to include other technologies such as biotechnology. The new focus directed attention to the interaction between humans and these technologies. The legal, ethical, social, and political impacts of these technologies on the individual, the health care professional, and society are also examined. The third change was the inclusion of a health care informatics specialty in the Master's Degree program. This specialty allowed nurses to obtain informatics degrees in areas of decision support systems or health communications. Lastly, the School of Nursing made a commitment to provide seamless curriculum that made learning opportunities accessible to a growing part-time student population regardless of geographic location or time boundaries. To this end, the School of Nursing began developing an on-line Master's program for its population-focused specialties including health care informatics.

Given these new and exciting changes in both UCHSC-SON and Hogeschool Holland, there was fertile ground to begin the next phase of this international exchange. The next phase spearheaded efforts to create an international course, co-developed by both schools of nursing. Both schools agreed that a web-based course was feasible and would further identify additional exchanges among faculty and students. The current web-based platform at UCHSC provided a solid foundation for the co-development of a specific international course. The pilot course emphasized Nursing Language and Classification Systems. This topic was selected because structuring data is relevant to nurses across the globe and work is being conducted in many countries. In the field of nursing informatics, the importance of a structured vocabulary is viewed as a necessary precondition for the retrieval and use of nursing data to make data-driven decisions. The structured vocabulary provides not only a means for nurses to communicate with each other and other disciplines; it provides an opportunity to make visible the process of nursing. This process of informatting is an important step in supporting theory-guided, evidence-based practice. A joint meeting held in Holland allowed for the development of the course. There were four units developed for this pilot. These units (The Importance of Structuring Nursing Phenomena; European Classification Efforts, American Classification Efforts; and Setting an International Research Agenda) were spread across a 9-week time period. The outcome competencies for this course were as follows. Upon completion of the course, the learner would be able to:

1. Articulate the importance of codifying nursing phenomena for nursing practice, administration, research, and informatics.
2. Explain the most commonly used system(s) in one's country.
3. Formulate strategies to foster the use of classification systems in their organizations.
4. Identify research initiatives from an international perspective.

The underlying method to reach these outcome competencies was to create a Learning Circle for an online course using the WebCT™ platform (Skiba, Springer, van Doeveren, & Walker, submitted for publ.). Students had an opportunity to dialogue about nursing in the context of their own countries and to discover that nursing speaks a common language regardless of country, native language, or culture. Students had an opportunity for a multicultural experience through the Learning Circle. The Learning Circle created a collaborative learning environment that would stimulate an international exchange between the student groups. The concept of *Learning Circle* was based upon the work of Riel (1994) and refered to "small electronic communities that form to accomplish specific goals". Riel (1994) designed a global education project through the use of learning circles. Students and instructors from several classrooms located around the world form a learning circle to accomplish a common goal. In this case, our common goal was to learn about the importance of Nursing Language and Classification Systems from a global perspective. According to Riel (1994), learning circles like quality circles, involved both participatory management and collective construction by participants. Instructors served as guides to facilitate learning and each learning circle constructed their own learning and shared it with other circles. Electronic community-based projects were shared with global partners as a way to make Nursing Language and Classification Systems more concrete and realistic within the context of one' s own country.

According to Riel (1994), there are six phases of the learning circle. We adapted these phases for this module. Here are the phases and their interpretation for this project:

1. Getting ready (Reviewing materials & gaining web-based competencies).
2. Opening the circle (Welcoming participants & introducing each circle. Unit 1 facilitates the opening of circles).
3. Planning circle projects (Assignments were designed to facilitate circles).
4. Exchanging student work. (Each learning circle took responsibility to teach one another about classification & language projects in their country.)
5. Organizing the circle final project. (Each circle will contribute

to establishing an international research agenda for nursing language and classification systems.)
6. Closing the circle. (Upon completion of the final project, learners will share closing remarks and participate in an evaluation of the learning circle project.)

Four course modules were created using a standard template developed by the UCHSC School of Nursing. The template consisted of the following items for each module: An introduction, outcome competencies for the module, readings, a learning guide, learning activities, competency evaluation, and faculty contact. The learning guide serves as the major vehicle for faculty to foster students learning in the module. The learning guide contained the faculty's pearls of wisdom, guidance on how to approach the module, clarifications of muddiest points or gray areas, hyperlinks to necessary resources, and overall strategies for learning. Here are some samples from the first module on the Importance of Structuring Nursing Phenomena.

Sample: Introduction
In the field of nursing informatics, the importance of a structured vocabulary is viewed as a necessary precondition for the retrieval and use of nursing data to make data-driven decisions. The structured vocabulary provides not only a means for nurses to communicate with each other and other disciplines; it provides an opportunity to make visible the process of nursing. This process of informatting or making nursing visible is important if nursing wants to support a theory-guided evidence-based practice. This unit introduces the basic concepts of health care terminology and structured vocabularies. The importance of structured vocabularies and classification systems are highlighted from numerous health care perspectives. This unit examines the basic principles to structure data so it is retrievable to make meaningful decisions and contribute to the development of nursing knowledge.

The introduction served to set the stage for the module and place the outcome competencies within the context of the entire course. A sample of first module's competencies is provided below.

Sample—Module 1: Outcome Competencies
Upon completion of the module, learners will be able to summarize the importance of codifying nursing phenomena for nursing practice, administration, research, and informatics.

Readings for each module were a combination of articles from both American and international journals and books. Whenever possible, readings available in English and Dutch were selected. The course made every effort to select articles available on-line or through the electronic library at the UCHSC. Full-text articles for over 50 journals were available through the UCHSC Library. All students were required to complete newly created on-line forms to obtain an electronic library card to access these resources.

Sample Readings:

Clark, J. & Lang, N. (1992). Nursing's next advance: An international classification for nursing practice. *International Nursing Review, 39*(4), 109–112.

Duisterhout, J. S., de Vries Robbe, P. F., van der Maas, A. A. F., with contribution of A. T. McCray (1997). Coding and classification. In J. H. van Bemmel & M. A. Musen (Eds.), *Handbook of Medical Informatics*. Heidelberg, Germany: Springer-Verlag.

Lang, N. (1995). *Nursing data systems: The emerging framework.* Washington, D.C.: American Nurses Association Publishing. Chapter 1 & 2, 11.

McCormick, K., & Jones, C. (September 30, 1998). Is one taxonomy needed for health care vocabularies and classifications? *Online Journal of Issues in Nursing, http://www.nursingworld. org/ojin/tpc7/tpc7_2.htm.*

Mortensen, R., Mantas, J., Manuela, M, Sermeus, W., Nielsen, G.H., & McAvinue, E. (1994). Telematics for health care in the European Union. In S. J. Grobe & E.S.P. Pluyter-Wenting (Eds.), *Nursing Informatics: An International Overview for Nursing in a Technological Era.* Amsterdam: Elsevier.

Saba, V. K. (pre-publication). Nursing information technology: Classification and management. Reprinted with permission.

Thompson, C. (1996). Research to support holistic nursing taxonomies. *Holistic Nursing Practice, 11*(1), 31–30.

Each module clearly defined the learning activities and gave learners a variety of tools to use for communication and presentations. For each module, assessment of competencies were clearly defined using critical elements. In the sample below, the critical elements for participation in on-line dialogues were clearly explicated.

Sample Competency Evaluation with Critical Elements

I. Facilitate a dialogue with your colleagues and guest lecturers about the classification efforts in a particular country. The critical elements of this dialogue include:
   a. Dialogue is collaborative: Two or more sides work together toward a common understanding.
   b. The goal is to find common ground in the dialogue.
   c. In dialogue, one listens to one side(s) in order to understand, find meaning, and find agreement.
   d. Dialogue causes introspection of one's own position.
   e. Dialogue assumes that many people have pieces of the answer and that together they can put them into a workable solution.

Several guest virtual faculty were asked to interact with students through the computer mediated conferencing tool provided by our web platform, WebCT™. The guest faculty included: Nicholas Hardiker, Research Fellow at the University of Manchester, Great Britain; Derek Hoy, Research Fellow at Glasgow Calendonian University, Scotland; William Goossen, Faculty at Leeuwarden Polytechnic, the Netherlands, Dr. Virginia Saba, Faculty at the Uniformed Service University, Dr. Suzanne Beyea, Research Co-Director, American Operating Room Nurses Association, and Dr. Amy Barton, Associate Dean for Practice at the University of Colorado.

An extensive evaluation was conducted to examine the results of the Learning Circle Project. There were three major components of the evaluation. The first component used an evaluation tool to assess the *Best Practices in Teaching and Learning in Web-based Nursing* courses. This tool is part of a benchmarking study being conducted by Indiana University, University of Kansas Medical Center, and University of Colorado Schools of Nursing (Billings, Skiba, Connors, & Zuniga, 1999). This tool, available on-line, allows students to assess outcomes (learning, socialization, satisfaction, preparation for real world work), educational practices (active learning, collaborative interactions) and technology experience (Billings et al., 1999). The second evaluation component was a measure of Social Presence. The social presence tool, developed by Gunawardena and Zittle (1997), consisted of 14 items used to embody the concept of immediacy. This concept included the perceived sense of an "online community" and the degree of social comfort with computer-mediated communication (CMC). The third evaluation component was an on-line semi-structured interview exploring the students' lived experiences with participation in a web-based course. Results of this evaluation will be reported at the Nursing Informatics 2000 International Conference (Skiba, Holloway, & Springer, 2000).

SUMMARY

In summary, there are four primary principles that can guide the development of collaborative international efforts. The first principle is to allow ample time for both faculty and students to develop collegial relationships before embarking on required assignments. Students and faculty need to feel comfortable with each other and need to work through language and cultural differences before trying to participate in a collaborative learning experience. This means building time into the course for students and faculty to dialogue.

The second principle is to insure that the relationship between schools is truly collaborative and thus teaching materials and learning activities meet the needs of both student groups. It is important that integrity of each program is maintained and that the collaboration reflects the shared values of both schools.

The third principle is to insure that the collaboration moves to an institutional partnership that is supported and nurtured by both organizations. Although the initial relationship may be between two colleagues, the wealth and the diversity of the institutions help to maintain and strengthen the partnership. As with all partnerships, there must be a commitment from both parties to create a shared vision and strategies to support the implementation of this vision.

The last principle is that this partnership must be fun and contribute to a learning experience. This partnership should create an atmosphere of excitement about learning and sharing. The diverse and rich experiences brought to the table by each partner must be valued and create a learning environment that allows both faculty and learners to grow and thrive.

REFERENCES

Aarts, J. (1989). A postgraduate program in nursing informatics. In L. C. Kingsland (Ed.). *Proceedings of the thirteenth annual symposium on computer applications in medical care,* 773–775.

Billing, D. , Skiba, D., Connors, H., & Zuniga, R. (1999). *Best practices in teaching and learning in web-based nursing courses.* Unpublished Benchmarking Study.

Chambers, M. (1994). Information technology and the curriculum. In P. Wainwright (Ed.), *Nursing informatics.* Edinburgh: Churchill Livingstone.

Graves, J., & Corcoran, S. (1989). The study of nursing informatics. *Image, 21*(4), 227–231.

Gunawardena, C., & Zittle, F. (1997). Social presence as a predictor of satisfaction within a computer-mediated conferencing environment. *American Journal of Distance Education, 11*(3), 8–26.

Peterson, H., & Gerdin-Jerlag, U. (Eds.) (1988). *Preparing nurses for using information systems: Recommended informatics competencies.* New York: National League for Nursing Press.

Riel, M. (1994). Global education through learning circles. In L. Harasim (Ed.). *Global networks: Computers and international communication* (p. 223). Cambridge: MIT Press.

Romano, C., & Heller, B. (1988). A curriculum model for graduate specialization in nursing informatics. In R.A. Greenes (Ed.)., *Proceedings of the twelfth annual symposium on computer applications in medical care,* 343–349.

Ronald, J. (1979). Computers and undergraduate nursing education: A report of an experimental introductory course. *Journal of Nursing Education, 18*(9), 4–9.

Ronald, J. (1991). A collaborative model for specialization in nursing informatics. In E. J. S. Hovenga, K. J. Hannah, K. A. McCormick, & J. S. Ronald (Eds.), Nursing informatics 91: Proceedings of the fourth international conference on nursing use of computers and information science (pp. 662–666). Heidelberg-Berlin, Germany: Springer-Verlag.

Ronald, J., & Skiba, D. (1987). *Guidelines for basic computer education in nursing.* New York: National League for Nursing Press.

Saranto, K. (1998). Outcomes of education in information technology at nursing polytechnics. *Health Informatics Journal, 4*(2), 84–91.

Skiba, D., Holloway, N., & Springer, H. (2000). Measurement of best practices and social presence in a Web-based international nursing informatics pilot course. In Saba, V. Carr, R. Sereus, W. Rocha, P. (Eds.), One Step beyond: The Evolution of Technology and Nursing. New Zealand: Adis International.

Skiba, D., & Mirque, D. (1994). The electronic community: An alternative health care approach. In S. Grobe & E.S.P. Pluyter-Wenting (Eds.), *Nursing informatics: An international overview for nursing in a technologic era.* Amsterdam, Netherlands: Elsevier Science.

Skiba, D., Simpson, R., & Ronald, J. (1992). HealthQuest/HBO Nurse Scholars program: A corporate partnership with nursing education. In J. Arnold & G. Pearson (Eds.), *Computer applications in nursing education and practice.* New York: National League for Nursing Press.

Skiba, D., & Springer, H. (1995). Computer-mediated learning experiences spanning the globe: A pilot study between schools of nursing in the USA and the Netherlands. In R. A. Greenes, H. E. Peterson, & D. J. Protti (Eds.), *Proceedings of the eighth world congress on medical informatics. International Medical Informatics Association.* Edmonton, Canada: HealthCare Computing & Communications Canada.

Skiba, D., Springer, H., van Doeveren, K., & Walker, P. H. (Submitted for publication). Learning Circle: An International Nursing Web Course.

11

Structuring a Knowledge Base: The arcs© Model

Judith Graves

This chapter is written as a case study to illustrate how an informatics program of research can be conducted. As such, it illustrates the initiation of the research program, the theoretical underpinnings, the proof of concept, and the many applications stemming from the research that help to evaluate and externally validate the theory and its implementation.

BEGINNINGS: HOW RESEARCH PROGRAMS ARISE

A research program is like a doctoral dissertation. It requires discipline and persistence as well as knowledge and skill. For this researcher, it requires a burning desire to answer a question to its fullest. The question which led to the *arcs©* research program arose when the author was a baccalaureate nursing student and found that research was indexed by key words and not by variables studied together. This was a bother throughout a career as a student, as a practitioner, and as an educator. Indexers at the National Library of Medicine rarely use the results section of the research report and *research findings* themselves are not indexed at all by any of the bibliographic indexing services (Horowitz, Fuller, Gillman, Stowe, & Weiner, 1982). While writing a doctoral dissertation, a commercial punch-hole card method was found that could be used to keep track of the supporting literature. In this method, a bibliographic citation was recorded along with the names of variables studied together and other pertinent information about the research. In the index, each different variable name was assigned a unique index number. One could then separate all the citation cards that contained information about a particular variable. It was fairly easy to re-sort the resulting cards for studies that contained information about pairs or sets of variables. A model of variables studied together could then be rather easily conceptualized. It was not until postdoctoral study in medical informatics that the tools for computerizing this methodology were found.

NEXT STEPS IN DEVELOPING AN INFORMATICS PROGRAM OF RESEARCH: THEORY AND PROOF OF CONCEPT

Given a research question, the next step in this research program was to develop the underlying theory. In this case, it was to define the structure of research knowledge and to explicate components that would be necessary for both indexing and modeling knowledge. Further, in informatics research, the theory would need to be implemented in a system to "prove" the concept—to show that the concept could work as expected.

THE STRUCTURE OF EMPIRICAL KNOWLEDGE: THE ONTOLOGY

Building a computerized system to index or model knowledge requires several things. First, it requires understanding the structure of the knowledge. Although not commonly referred to in the informatics literature as *ontology* at that time, the study of knowledge structures was and is considered legitimate and necessary for developing decision support systems and computational languages. Since the program was to be built within a database management program, the structure was needed to develop the logical model for the database (tables, relations, and data fields). Second, for the model to be of general use, it needed to be verified that the knowledge structure is applicable across disciplines.

The commonality of a definition of scientific (empirical) knowledge across sciences was quickly verified from textbooks in science and research theory and methods. Briefly, scientific knowledge is considered across sciences to be the (numerical) relationship (the finding, the result) between two or more variables studied together under given conditions (including design and methods of analysis).

This definition provides the major set of elements and the relationships between them. A careful study of research reports from the literature of nursing and reference disciplines was needed, however, to understand the expression of this structure in the various health science disciplines and to verify that, despite some vocabulary differences, major concepts were understandable across disciplines. This too was verification of the obvious: nurses universally read research from various disciplines and, while the content may not be well understood, there is no difficulty understanding the use of the research concepts. The benefit of the study was to get a grasp of the detail of the knowledge structure and the variety needed across disciplines and domains. This early work on the structure and modeling of empirical knowledge is reported in Graves, 1990.

The data fields identified to express a unit of research knowledge and the relationships between the structural elements can be considered the ontology of empirical research knowledge. Inter-discipline and even intra-discipline differences in expression of a unit of knowledge lie not in the major structural elements or relationships between them but rather in the various vocabulary terms and typologies used to instantiate the various elements. For example, some will prefer to use one typology of research designs, others will another. These are instantiation issues and do not affect the ontological structure itself: *all empirical research has a defined design type.*

IMPLEMENTATION IN A COMPUTER PROGRAM: PROOF OF CONCEPT

The ontology was implemented in a computer program first called ARKS (Graves, 1990) and renamed later as *arcs©*. As it currently exists, this program provides a structured set of data fields needed to fully describe units of empirical knowledge. The implementation is considered a knowledgebase rather than a database because not only are units of knowledge retrievable *as* units of knowledge but because the units of knowledge can be used computationally to solve various problems. The major structural elements are: Source > Study > Knowledge. The relationships between them are hierarchical (one to many).

At its simplest, the program allows a scientist to organize and track information about the scientific literature. One of the main uses of the ontology is to gather data by which to build scientific models:

concept maps and theoretical knowledge models. Given the names of variables studied together and the statistical relationship between them, *arcs©* aggregates the knowledge from all studies in the knowledgebase. Using a single unconditional rule of logic, *arcs©* then generates a relational model of all relationships between a user-selected focal variable and all variables studied directly with it. Tables summarizing the findings accompany each graphical model so the user can make inclusion/exclusion decisions about various relationships and so the findings can be added to the model to show a true knowledge model, rather than just a concept model. Right now, the addition of findings to the map is manual. One version of *arcs©* also models two additional levels of indirect relationships as well as the direct relationships. The causal/associational knowledge models provide significant decision support to clinicians and other appraisers "weighing evidence" for practice, researchers building theoretical models for testing, and theorists for building and comparing literature-based models of knowledge.

Validity of the ontology

arcs© was implemented on several different platforms using different relational database management system shells over the last 12 years. The program was used by colleagues and students in such diverse domains of research as menstrual cycle research (Robinson, 1989), predictive and structural variables related to metabolic energy expenditure in traumatic brain injury (Sunderland, Graves, Heilbrun, 1990), caregiver burden research (Boyd, 1989 and Maurin, & Boyd, 1990). Except for the addition of detail, the ontology has remained stable across disciplines and users. It is not nursing specific but, rather, is sufficiently general for empirical research across disciplines. The cross-discipline and cross-domain applicability provides external validity for the ontology.

EVALUATION OF THE RESEARCH PROGRAM: USES OF THE ONTOLOGY

Instantiation of the ontology for nursing research

For nursing science specifically, the ontology has been used as the matrix within which to develop a nursing research classification system . . . the set of values that instantiate the ontology specifically for nursing research (NRCS©[1]). The ontology together with the classification system provides the logical model for the database that serves the Registry of Nursing Research©[2]. Although researchers are not currently asked to provide values for all data elements in the classification system, the underlying database would permit such detail. Implementation of the database model of *arcs*© and the NRCS© differ slightly to accommodate different purposes. However, data can be mapped between the two systems.

The research classification system (as well as the ontology) is thought to be widely applicable throughout the health sciences with but minor vocabulary changes to suit the vocabulary preferences of various disciplines. For example, one version of the *arcs*© program uses the Sigma Theta Tau Nursing Research Classification System© for default instantiation values for all possible fields and another version has no default values: a user has to build his/her own controlled vocabulary to instantiate the database.

Cross-discipline applicability will also require some added detail to provide the different depths of data detail important to various disciplines. For example, the NRCS does not contain much descriptive detail about randomized controlled trial design because, at the time it was designed, there were few of these trials being done in nursing and even fewer registered with the Virginia Henderson International Nursing Library. Nonetheless, this is an issue of depth of instantiation, not a structural issue—the structural element, research design, for this detail is explicit in the ontology.

Indexing the scientific literature

Using the ontology, a new paradigm for indexing research has been implemented in a working system. This has ramifications for nursing science and science generally. Findings (aka knowledge) are indexed by variable name or research concept in the Registry of Nursing Research© in the Virginia Henderson International Nursing Library of Sigma Theta Tau International (STTI) (http://www.stti.iupui.edu/

---

[1] © Nursing Research Classification System, 1994 to present held by Sigma theta Tau International.

[2] © Registry of Nursing Research, 1994 to present held by Sigma Theta Tau International.

library > Registry). Researchers submit the names of variables studied together (together with other study details). This index is a content vocabulary of nursing research—the *things in the world* that are studied in all clinical domains of nursing. Indexes of practice knowledge are still in the planning stage.

In addition to the Registry Index, the Virginia Henderson International Library has two other indexes formed by variable names: a) the HIV/AIDS Knowledgebase using arcs© software, identifies the vocabulary of variables studied in the clinical practice domain of HIV/AIDS between 1985 and 1998 (http://www.stti. iupui.edu/library > Knowledgebases > arcs Knowledgebases > HIV/AIDS, and b) the Index of Nursing Research Knowledge (http://www.stti.iupui.edu/library > Knowledge Indexes > Nursing Research).

The variable names in the indexes of each of the three knowledge resources are at different levels of abstraction: the *arcs©* variables list of independent and dependent variables represent the operational level of the variable, the name of the entities that are specifically measured (operationalized) in the studies. The Registry Index of findings also includes some variable names identified at the operational level. These are the names submitted by the researchers themselves. When library staff identify the study variables, they must be identified from the abstracts. Variables in abstracts are generally named at a higher level of abstraction than the operational level. At least one level more generalized (abstracted) than the operational level.

The operational-level variable names and their abstractions form *a natural thesaurus of nursing research*, evolving naturally from research studies rather than being conceptually organized, as are most bibliographic thesauri (CINAHL, MeSH). The value of this is limited by the lack of availability of both levels of the variable name in the sources of the vocabulary. The *arcs©* knowledgebase builders use author-defined abstractions when possible, thus making both the operational level of the variable and the abstraction available at the same time. There is, however, no way to know for sure whether the author assigned the abstraction or whether the knowledgebase builder assigned it. Further, many of the same terms will be abstracted differently by the researchers, and vice versa, thus making the thesaurus less accurate in searching and retrieving information. Perhaps the truest value of this natural research thesaurus lies in its representation of the natural structure of nursing knowledge.

Terms introduced via the automated indexing process of the Nursing Research Index which covers the 30+ research-specific and clinical nursing journals containing the highest proportion of research articles do include variable names as well as other research-relevant terms from the abstract. This Index, as it stands today, is least representative of nursing's research vocabulary in that terms that are not study variables at all are included in the index along with variables. Further, the variables tend to be named at one or more levels of abstraction than the operational variable. Automating the separation of the actual variable names to include in the nursing research vocabulary is underway at the Library.

Knowledge Retrieval

Despite the more general nature of the Research Knowledge Index, or perhaps because of it, the contribution to improve retrieval of knowledge from the health science literature is considerable. The largely automated methodology for generating this Index was developed by Dr. John Weiner, epidemiologist and informaticist, of 24th Century Press. Weiner, like Graves, started from a position of identifying variables studied together to index the scientific literature. Deciding that automating the variable name identification process using automated information processing methods applied to the scientific literature was not feasible, Weiner developed an automated information-processing strategy based on identifying salient linked terms in sentences of research abstracts. The pragmatic value of Weiner's and Graves' approaches, however, lies in the improvement in search accuracy for knowledge retrieval. As does the linkage between variables studied together, the linkage between terms linked in sentences of the research abstract sets a context that is missing in single-term key word searching algorithms.

Concern for vocabulary

The concern for research vocabulary goes beyond the ability to objectively document nursing's science focus, interesting as that is. Most nurses cannot leave their stations to go to the library like professionals in other disciplines. We need to find ways to bring nursing *knowledge* (findings) to the point of care. With the hope of automating the clinical record comes the hope of linking research knowledge to the client record directly and automatically. The clinical information system and the knowledge system must then be able to talk to one another. Vocabulary is crucial to this communication. It is probable that salient linkages between vocabulary terms will improve the accuracy of the communication between systems, just as they improve retrieving knowledge in the first place.

The reader is reminded that it is the *knowledge* that needs to be linked to the record, NOT a listing of author, citation, index terms, and abstracts. Thus the preferred linkage uses actual variables studied together as the index to actual findings. Improved accuracy will depend on knowing how the variables are operationally defined in order to link vocabulary terms accurately. Additional information may be desirable to ensure population relevance. Of course, the most desirable situation would be an illumination of all conditioning factors affecting the knowledge to ensure an appropriate match between patient/client and the research knowledge. The technology needed to implement both knowledge retrieval and to determine fit of research population and conditions to study patients conditions is already available via the *arcs©* program and the Registry of Nurse Researchers at the Virginia Henderson International Nursing library.

The next issue is whether or not the clinical record and the research literature can "talk" to each other. Research is now underway to examine the co-occurrence of vocabulary terms between relevant vocabulary systems. Dr. Marcelline Harris, postdoctoral fellow in Health Informatics at the University of Minnesota, Rochester, leads this work. Co-investigators are multidisciplinary (nursing research, nursing informatics, medical informatics). Semantics and representation within various data modeling approaches will be studied. The most important aspect of this work will be to define and delimit the problem of linking research to the clinical record.

NEXT QUESTIONS IN THE *ARCS©* RESEARCH PROGRAM

How can arcs© better support decision making?

Some improvements concern the ease with which *arcs©* supports decision making. These improvements involve automating what must now be done manually. The next stage of research for the *arcs©* program is the automation of these strategies. First is to automate the conditioning of theoretical models within the modeling program itself. Currently, the user must delimit the model manually using desired criteria or by pre-building a sub-knowledgebase in which the conditions are applied and modeling the sub-knowledgebase.

Weighting evidence for practice using a given and customizable set of criteria (research design, power, and significance parameters, etc.) would be another application of improved condition-based knowledge modeling. This too, can be done manually in the current version using user-supplied criteria.

Can *arcs©* be used computationally for evaluating and proposing new theory?

The name, *arcs©*, comes from graph theory where an arc is composed of two nodes connected by a line. Digraph theory adds the potential for directionality of the line—a perfect model for empirical knowledge. It has been suggested by a computer scientist colleague that Warshall's algorithm in graph theory be used to automate identification of gaps and conflicts in knowledge matrices (Aho, Hopcroft, & Ullman, 1983; Walker & Avant, 1995) and demonstrate a visual matrix-based method for comparing relationships in model building. Addition of computational ability to *arcs©* to automate the manual matrix work may someday provide a methodology for postulating new theories, critiquing theories, thus leading to the discovery of new knowledge.

What methods can be used to improve data and knowledge acquisition?

Data acquisition.

Thus far, all the data entered into *arcs©* except for source information available from bibliographic databases must be obtained and entered into the program by the user. A program to automate moving data between other databases and file systems will encourage scientists to move research data they already have into *arcs©* to take advantage of the indexing and modeling properties of the program. This is a step in improving *data acquisition* for the program.

The surge of structured abstracts in the health science literature holds some promise for automating entry of data about the research study itself. Work to process the narrative descriptions of these abstracts into more specific data values of the research classification system is needed to create a database of study descriptors for comparing studies and determining relevance to one's clinical purpose.

Knowledge acquisition.

More importantly, but also more difficult, is to find ways to automate the identification of variable names and relationships (and other selected data) and findings from research studies so they can be imported into *arcs©*: a knowledge acquisition problem. A manual method of harvesting knowledge that is expressed in numeric relationship displays such as tables and graphs is relatively fast, taking only 5–10 minutes per article. Knowledge embedded in narrative text takes closer to an hour to locate, verify, and enter.

In an ideal world, we would learn how to process natural language and let the computer do the work. Years of effort in this area have resulted in important improvements but have not led to the kind of accuracy needed to link research knowledge to the patient record.

Partial informatics solutions exist now. The cleanest and the most accurate is to have researchers register their own research such as is done in the Registry of the Virginia Henderson International Nursing Library. This is a radical change in the traditional research paper–based narrative publishing paradigm and requires significant education of and behavioral change by researchers. As Homer Warner has been heard to say, medical informatics *is* a behavioral science.

Second in accuracy is using the research-abstract processing algorithm developed by John Weiner and post-process the resulting files to eliminate terms that do not represent measured variables and therefore do not link directly to findings. Methods for post-processing to identify variables only are under study at the Virginia Henderson International Library.

There are drawbacks to processing abstracts, however. To build knowledge models and work with them computationally, one needs the names of the operational level variables not provided by processing abstracts. As explained earlier, variable names in abstracts are usually at least one level of abstraction away from the operational definition. So while this method has great promise for providing better indexing of the scientific literature, it is not too promising for knowledge acquisition for *arcs©* if one wishes to use the program for building knowledge models.

Beyond vocabulary issues

Given that we can link research terms to terms in the clinical record accurately and match population and environmental characteristics of the research and the patient of concern, how do we decide which research is of sufficient *quality* to link. How do we determine quality? Can we computationally evaluate conflicting evidence and gaps in knowledge as might be done by *arcs©*? Could we use this evidence together with the closeness of "fit" between the patient situation and the research study conditions to provide a measure of confidence in actually applying the knowledge clinically? Is it enough to provide the links and let the clinician make the relevance and applicability decisions?

SUMMARY

This chapter serves as a long-needed update of the research program into empirical knowledge structures and knowledge modeling. It is written with the informatics student in mind so that it also serves as a case study for those learning how to do (or not do) informatics research. Although it is not a formal report of research, close attention is paid to the research questions asked and answered and the use of evaluation using application success.

Author's commentary on the state of nursing informatics research

In this researcher's opinion, there are two significant hindrances to progress in nursing informatics. Funding from nursing must improve. The work described here has been entirely privately funded[3] ... a situation which has significantly delayed development and testing.

[3] Gratitude is expressed to an anonymous donor who contributed to the program via the College of Nursing at the University of Utah, the George S. Delores Dore' Eccles Foundation, and the Helene Fuld Foundation for funding of the arcs© research.

Only after 15 or 16 years is the work to a point that the effects of direct access to knowledge on patient care and outcomes or the use of knowledge models in planning intervention strategies can be studied. Much nursing informatics research will of necessity be similarly constrained because it involves long stages of building proof of concept applications and testing them in various environments and for different purposes. These efforts must be supported by agencies such as the National Institute of Nursing Research.

Moreover, nursing needs to accept responsibility for evaluating and funding nursing informatics research. Medical informatics research is not nursing informatics research. Nursing practice is different from medical practice and systems to each must be responsive to these differences. Therefore, nursing must fund its own work in building systems to support nursing practice. For example, the research on vocabulary described above will be severely hindered by the fact that nursing continues to have inadequate clinical information systems that contain atomic level data patient observations. In my opinion, this is a result of inadequate funding of nursing informatics research designed to build clinical nursing information systems, not a lack of sound nursing informatics research proposals.

Solutions to the problem. The nursing informatics researcher has not and probably will not be able to count on the type of federal funding that helped develop and test well-known clinical medical information systems and expert decision support systems. We must work first in the laboratory environment. Both students and faculty in the nursing informatics programs are much more able to use computers to model their ideas without having to depend on programmers and medical informatics students. Clinical data sets of atomic level patient observations can be built from records when not available from real systems. A few "real" systems are appearing; and the agencies might be willing to part with data for use in a nursing informatics laboratory situation. I encourage you to not only enjoin the battles but also to work around them until others see the light as we do.

Despite these difficulties, sound nursing informatics research can be done and is well worth the effort to those interested in the field. To be on the leading edge of change in knowledge is in the soul of all researchers. To be on the leading edge of change in technology as well as knowledge that will improve patient care is available only to the nursing informatics researcher. To me, there is nothing that is professionally more rewarding.

REFERENCES

Aho, A. V., Hopcroft, J. E., & Ullman, J. D. (1983). *Data structures and algorithms.* Reading Massachusetts: Addison-Wesley Publishing Co.

Boyd, C. (1989). Caregiver burden concept analysis. Unpublished paper presented at the Western Institute of Nursing Conference, Salt Lake City, UT.

Graves, J. R. (1990). A research knowledge system (ARCS) for storing, managing and modeling knowledge from the scientific literature. *Advances in Nursing Science, 13*(2).

Horowitz, R. S., Fuller, S. S. Gilman, N. J., Stowe, S. M., & Weiner, J. M. (1982). Concurrence in content descriptions: Author versus medical subject headings (MeSH). *Proceedings of the American Society of Information Science,* (19), 139–140.

Maurin, J. T., & Boyd C. B. (1990). Burden of mental illness on the family: a critical review. *Archives of Psychiatric Nursing, 4*(2), 99–107.

Robinson, C. (1989). "Relationship of menstrual cycle variables: Research and utilization." Poster presented at the 8th Conference of the Society for Menstrual Cycle Research, Salt Lake City, UT.

Sunderland, P. M., Graves, J. R., & Heilbrun, M. P. (1990, Winter). Evaluation of the efficiency and accuracy of computerized domain analysis in critical nutrition in traumatic brain injury. Unpublished paper presented at the annual Richard Linde Neurosurgery Conference, Snowbird, UT.

Walker, L., & Avant, K. C. (1995). *Strategies for theory construction in nursing* (3rd Edition). Norwalk, CT: Appleton & Lange.

12

Telehealth and Nursing
Carole A. Gassert

Telehealth is one of the areas of health care that will grow tremendously within the next decade. It will radically change the way nurses' practice. To most nurses the future of telehealth practice is very exciting, others who are reluctant to change or who feel challenged by using technology, may view telehealth less favorably. This chapter will define and describe telehealth practice, discuss issues of using telehealth technologies, and identify potential funding sources to expand telehealth practice for nursing.

WHAT IS TELEHEALTH?

In 1977, the term telehealth was used to describe the use of electronic communication and information technologies to support a wide variety of health activities (Conrad, 1977). Telecommunication technologies are used to transmit video, audio, images, text, signals, or signs through an electronic system such as a telephone, facsimile, video-phone, computer, video conferencing, or interactive television systems. In addition to telemedicine services, telehealth activities include the health education of communities, the education of health professionals, public health research, and the administration of health services. The term telehealth is significant because it expands the concept of delivery of services at a distance and implies a broader range of activities than are traditionally covered by what has been called telemedicine.

[1] The views expressed in this paper are solely those of the author and not necessarily those of the Health Resources and Services Administration, Department of Health and Human Services.

Telemedicine is defined as the use of electronic communication and information technologies to provide clinical care at a distance (Office of Rural Health Policy, 1997; Institute of Medicine, 1996). A 1999 survey of 249 telemedicine programs in the United States indicates the most common clinical care offered through telemedicine are radiology, dermatology, cardiology, and psychiatry. Less frequently used clinical applications are emergency services, home health, pathology, and oncology (Dakins, 1999).

The Healthcare Financing Administration (HCFA) uses the term telemedicine to mean the use of telecommunications to furnish medical information and services. HCFA states that consultation is provided through a two-way interactive process that includes both the patient and consultant and the use of audio and video equipment. In some instances, a store and forward technique can be used to transfer specified images, such as x-rays, computerized topography, and EKG interpretation. HCFA uses the American Medical Association (AMA) definition of consultation and states further that tele-consultation is simply a new way of delivering a consultation. Accordingly, HCFA requires that a patient be present during the consultation.

Our international colleagues have adopted another term, telematics, to describe telehealth practice. Telematics is considered to be a composite term that includes health-related activities, services, and systems, carried out over a distance using information and communication technologies. The purpose of telematics is to promote global health, control disease control, and provide health care, education, management, and research. Like the term telehealth, telematics includes tele-education, telemedicine, and health services research. In describing telematics, the concepts of lifelong learning, health promotion, participative education, education without frontiers, and continuing professional education are included.

To further complicate the description of telehealth practice some nurses have adopted the term telenursing to define the practice of nursing over distance using telecommunications technology , (ANA, 1997; Chaffee, 1999, NCSBN, 1996). Several years ago Senator Conrad cautioned against the use of terms that draw artificial distinctions that could slow the development and implementation of integrated systems within telehealth practice (Conrad, 1977).

This author believes that "telenursing" is such a term. Some nurses have stated that telenursing is a specialty and are pushing for certification as telenurses. But there has been no new domain of focus demonstrated; the domain of focus remains clinical nursing. Nurses engaged in telehealth practice simply are using tools to collect and exchange information needed about patients to deliver clinical care over a distance. These nurses must be adequately prepared to use telehealth tools; the same way cardiac intensive care nurses must be prepared to use an EKG or pressure monitor while delivering care.

The basis of reimbursement for telehealth practice presents another reason for avoiding the use of the term "telenursing." Currently, HCFA reimburses for telemedicine consultations for certain patient activity codes, that is, Current Procedural Codes (CPT). Some advanced practice nurses are eligible to participate in telemedicine consultations, but the regulations do not address telenursing.

More than half of the telehealth programs surveyed by Dakins reported that they do not currently emphasize better outcomes as a measurement of success (Dakins, 1999). It may be more beneficial, therefore, for nursing to demonstrate positive outcomes for nurses engaged in telehealth practice, than to try to argue for telenursing as a specialty.

HISTORY OF TELEHEALTH

Telehealth is not a new concept for delivering health care; it has existed for 50 years under the title of telemedicine. During that time, telehealth has gained, lost, and regained popularity as a system for increasing access to health care. Four early projects have been discontinued. Implemented during the 1950s, the Space Technology Applied to Rural Papago Advanced Health Care (STARPAHC) project provided care on the Papago Indian Reservation in Arizona. STARPAHC used a mobile van to connect providers and hospitals through microwave television and phone technology. The project lasted for 20 years.

In 1959, the University of Nebraska used closed circuit television to link remote psychiatric hospitals to large medical centers for consultation. This project lasted for 6 years. In 1968, the Massachusetts General Hospital used microwave television to link with the medical station at Boston's Logan Airport and the Veterans Administration Hospital in Bedford, MA. Before the project was discontinued, it was expanded to schools, courts, and prisons. In 1972, Mt. Sinai School of Medicine initiated a project that used closed circuit television to link nurse practitioners in a primary care clinic that served a large Hispanic population with the New York City Hospital.

Four telehealth projects implemented since 1986 seem to have overcome problems of sustainability and are ongoing. The Mayo Clinic Satellite Network was established in 1986. It has used satellites to link the Rochester, Minnesota campus with clinics in Scottsdale, Arizona and Jacksonville, Florida. The Texas Telemedicine Project, established in 1988, uses interactive video technology to link Austin and Giddings, Texas. This project was started without federal funding and has demonstrated costeffectiveness in delivering health care.

A second Texas project, the Texas Tech HealthNet, was started in 1989. Images are transmitted over phone lines, satellite uplinks, and facsimile machines to service the 500-mile area of rural western Texas. Perhaps the most widely known telehealth project was implemented in 1991, at the Medical College of Georgia. Academic and medical facilities are linked throughout the state in a system known as GSAMS.

The goals of telemedicine have been to overcome barriers of distance and time in delivering care. Equipment and regulatory challenges and lack of provider acceptance have hampered widespread adoption of telemedicine. More recently, however, interest has been rekindled by the digital convergence of technologies available for telehealth practice.

STATUS OF TELEHEALTH

During the later 1990s, the number of telehealth projects have increased dramatically, but it is impossible to determine the exact number of projects that currently exist. In 1995, the office of Rural Health Policy (ORHP), HRSA, contracted with Abt Associates and the University of Colorado to study telemedicine in rural America (ORHP, 1997). More than 95% of all 2472 non-Federal rural hospitals responded to the survey. There were 324 (13.8%) reported active telemedicine programs. More than two thirds of the programs offered only radiology services. Ninety-seven programs (29.9%) offered additional clinical services via telemedicine. Many of the telemedicine programs were in their first year of operation. Rural hospitals with telemedicine programs most frequently reported a capacity of 50 or less beds. More than half of the rural telemedicine received Federal finding.

In 1997, the Federal Telehealth Directory listed 187 projects that received Federal funding (HRSA, 1997). The total number increased by one in 1998 (HRSA, 1998). The 1999 directory is available on-line at *http://telehealth.hrsa.gov.*

When reviewing projects listed in the two available Federal directories, it is of concern that in 1997 only 26 grantees included nursing in the abstracts describing their projects. The number rose to 28 in 1998. Further analysis shows that six projects included advanced practice nurses and six projects included home care in 1997. Those numbers fell to four and five respectively in 1998. Five projects targeted continuing education projects for nurses in both 1997 and 1998. Nurse training (academic programs) as part of telemedicine projects rose from five in 1997 to seven in 1998. And finally delivery of nursing services increased from four in 1997 to seven in 1998. It is interesting that HRSA and the Rural Utilities Service each funded 10 projects that included nursing in 1997. HRSA funded a total of 16 projects with nursing included in 1998. Nursing was included in additional projects funded in 1998 by the National Telecommunication and Information Administration, National Library of Medicine, Appalachian Regional Commission, and HCFA. Although nursing may be included in additional projects but not listed in the abstract, these findings indicate that nursing in general has not collaborated with interdisciplinary health care providers to take advantage of federal funding opportunities in telehealth.

In 1998, the Science Advisory Board (SAB) conducted an on-line survey to understand trends affecting the use of telemedicine. SAB is a worldwide panel of about 4,000 life science and medical professionals from over 60 countries. More than 500 participants responded to the survey, but the exact number of telemedicine projects was unclear. Of those projects reported, most have been in existence for 1 to 2 years (31%) or 3 to 4 years (36%). Programs responded that they had implemented telemedicine to deliver quality care to rural and underserved areas (17%), to respond to increased demand for medical information (17%), and to meet the desire to enhance continuing education (15%). The most frequently reported clinical use of telehealth systems was for provider to provider clinical consultations.

Respondents cited patient confidentiality as the most common concern of using telemedicine (Telehealth Magazine, 1998).

Dakins mailed the third annual telehealth market survey to 249 telemedicine and teleradiology program managers who subscribe to *Telehealth Magazine* (formerly *Telemedicine and Telehealth Networks*) in 1999 (Dakins, 1999) compared to 296 subscribers in 1997 (Dakins, 1997). The question is whether this reflects a decrease in the number of telehealth programs or simply a decrease in the number of subscriptions to the journal. Dakins (1999) believes that telehealth attracts new enthusiasts and retains "old-timers." Telehealth adopters have consistently reflected a desire to increase access to care as the primary reason for implementing a telehealth program. Newer adopters also state a need to provide the highest quality service at the lowest cost.

The focus of telehealth services changed in 1999. Radiology and dermatology remained at the top of the list of services provided. However, cardiology rebounded from a decrease in use noticed the previous year. Emergency care, pathology, and oncology services all decreased as telehealth services provided over the past 2 years. Surprisingly, the provision of telehealth home health services, an area of interest to nurses (Dansky, Bowles, & Palmer, 1999; Sharp, 1998) decreased significantly from 27% to 17% in 1999 (Dakins, 1999).

Given the existence of predominantly new telehealth programs and a changing emphasis on services provided, one may ask whether telehealth programs have been evaluated to determine if there are quality programs within healthcare. Since 1996, *Telehealth Magazine* has acknowledged the top 10 programs in the United States. Five criteria used to select the top programs are:

- Program is designed to fulfill a defined clinical or healthcare delivery need;
- Program is self-supporting or sustainable without public funding;
- Organizational support for the program is evident through financial, administrative, or management maintenance.
- Services provided are accepted by physicians, allied healthcare providers, and patients.
- Program activities, costs, and outcomes are monitored (Dakins & Kincade, 1998).

Four sites have continually received top ratings for their programs and have received special recognition. These programs are University of Vermont/Fletcher Allen Health Care, Burlington; University of Texas Medical Branch, Galveston; Allina Health System, Minneapolis; and Texas Tech University/HealthNet, Lubbock (Kincade, 1999).

ISSUES IN TELEHEALTH PRACTICE

Even though exemplar telehealth programs exist, more widespread use of telehealth technologies is needed to increase patient access to care. Discussions about ways to increase use of telehealth technologies within health care include the following issues: reimbursement, licensure, security, provider acceptance, competence, and telecommunications costs. This author believes other key issues are the general separation of telehealth and informatics and need for evaluation data. Each of these issues will be addressed.

Reimbursement

Reimbursement for telehealth services has been a key issue for program expansion and survival. Some private insurers do reimburse for telehealth services, but the percentage remains quite small. The Abt study reported 8% of rural telemedicine programs had successfully negotiated reimbursement with private insurers (ORHP, 1997). At least four states, California, Oklahoma, Louisiana, and Texas, have passed laws that mandate reimbursement for telemedicine services. The California law indicates that telemedicine includes health care delivery, diagnosis, consultation, treatment, transfer of medical data, and education using interactive audio, video, or data communications. It does not include services delivered by phone or fax. Louisiana also excludes phone and fax from telemedicine services.

Medicaid law does not recognize telemedicine as a distinct service, each state has the option of whether or not to recognize it as a cost-effective alternative to more traditional ways of delivering medical care. To be accepted, telemedicine services must meet Federal requirements of efficiency, economy, and quality of care. Abt Associates (ORHP, 1997) reported that less than 25% of non-Federal rural telemedicine programs were successful in getting reimbursement for Medicaid patient telemedicine encounters.

States that do cover telemedicine do so in the form of physician consultation. Nonphysician practitioners are covered depending on their scope of practice. As of June, 2000, 17 states reimburse for telemedicine services for Medicaid patients. A current list of states that reimburse for telemedicine can be accessed through the HCFA web page at *http://www.hcfa.gov/medicaid/telelist.htm.*

HCFA has allowed limited reimbursement for telemedicine services to Medicare patients. Physicians have been reimbursed for telemedicine services provided in HCFA demonstration projects, for teleconsultation services delivered to patients in health professional shortage areas (HPSA) when face-to-face meetings were not required, and for teleradiology and long distance ECK and EEG interpretations. In the Abt study, less than 7% of non-Federal telemedicine projects were reimbursed for Medicare patients receiving services by telemedicine (ORHP, 1997).

The Balanced Budget Act of 1997 (BBA) has expanded reimbursement for telemedicine services provided to Medicare patients. In the HCFA rule issued October 7, 1998, several procedural codes were listed as being acceptable for reimbursement of telemedicine services for patients in HPSA. And for the first time, nurse practitioners, nurse midwives, and clinical nurse specialists are eligible for reimbursement as consulting practitioners. The reimbursement rule requires that an eligible practitioner present the patient to the consulting practitioner. Patients must also be present during the teleconsultation event.

Even though BBA was designed to increase reimbursement, many telehealth programs feel it is not inclusive enough to really benefit their programs. At a recent telehealth meeting, HRSA telehealth grantees stated that only 5% of all telemedicine events have actually been eligible for reimbursement under the current BBA rules (Tracey, 1999). Work is therefore underway to convince Congress to amend the BBA to allow all registered nurses to present patients during a consultation, to increase the allowable procedural codes to include outpatient follow-up activities that nurses more commonly perform, and to add store-and-forward technologies to those eligible for reimbursement.

Licensure

Increased sophistication and decreased cost of telehealth technologies has allowed many projects to cover even larger demographic areas. As the projects expand across state lines, the issues of interstate licensure have increased in importance. One of the issues is what constitutes interstate telehealth practice. There is growing agreement that real time videoconferencing, phone call centers, Internet, advanced decision support systems, and remote robotic procedures are examples of telehealth technologies and activities that when used across state lines constitute interstate practice (Waters, 1999). There is still disagreement, however, about changes that result from using telecommunications and how they have redefined interstate practice. For example, telecommunications has resulted in individualization of information, ambiguity between product and services, elimination of legal and geographic boundaries, expansion of consumer choice and elimination of time and space. Therefore, all of these outcomes of cyberspace have added to concern about what constitutes interstate practice.

A second licensure issue of growing concern is who has jurisdiction when telehealth technologies are used across state lines. Regulatory agencies have indicated that since the practice of medicine occurs in the state where the patient lives, physicians and nurses must hold valid licenses in all states where they deliver professional services. Exemptions to this ruling include emergencies, and physician to physician consultations that are not reimbursed and not documented.

Four solutions have been proposed for interstate practice. For physicians, the American Medical Association and American College of Radiology have recommended a full and unrestricted license for each state in which a provider delivers care through telehealth practice. As of October 1999, thirty-seven states and the District of Columbia have passed laws that require full and unrestricted licensure for physicians involved in interstate practice (Levy, 1999). This could add considerable expense to patient practices and discourage the use of telehealth to reach those patients who need it most.

Requiring a full and unrestricted license is contradictory to a 1996 recommendation by the Federation of Medical State Boards (FMSB), the regulatory organization for medical licensing boards. The FMSB model recommends issuance of a special purpose license (SPL) to cover interstate practice. The SPL is issued only if a physician has an unrestricted license in all states where he/she is licensed and receives a favorable response to a query of the FMSB Data Bank. The SPL brings a physician under the jurisdiction of the state in which an unrestricted, full license is held and under the jurisdiction of any and all states in which a SPL is held for the purpose of practicing across state lines. The SPL, like a full and unrestricted license, clarifies the jurisdiction of medical practice. Six states have passed legislation based on the FMSB model and nine additional states are considering adopting the model (Levy, 1999).

A third solution posed for interstate licensure is national standards and licensure. In 1998, the PEW Health Professions Commission indicated that health professions regulation is moving toward national standards (PEW, 1998). Some advocate a Federal role in national licensure that would leave the right to protect health and safety with the states. The Federal role has not been clearly identified, but it may be that of a catalyst to remove barriers to telehealth practice caused by licensure restrictions.

The nursing community has suggested a different solution for regulating interstate practice. In 1997, the National Council of State Boards of Nursing (NCSBN) Delegate Assembly agreed to promote a model of mutual recognition for registered nurses and licensed practical nurses in which nurses obtain a state-based license that is nationally recognized and locally enforced. Under mutual recognition, state boards of nursing agree to recognize the nursing licenses of other states through a compact, a legal document that regulates business between two or more states. In other words, the nurse obtains one license in the state of residence and can practice in other states that agree to participate in the compact without obtaining additional licenses. Nurses remain accountable for their practice according to the practice acts in states in which they are delivering services (Hutcherson & Williams, 1999).

To date, eleven states, Arkansas, Delaware, Iowa, Maryland, Mississippi, Nebraska, North Carolina, South Dakota, Texas, Utah, and Wisconsin, have passed the nursing compact. Additional states are planning to introduce the mutual recognition compact in upcoming legislation. The compact assigns jurisdiction for disciplinary actions to boards of nursing of both the residential state and the remote state, that is, the state where the nurse practices, but does not live.

Although the compact is being increasingly accepted in the nursing community, as evidenced by the introduction and passage of the compact within state legislatures, not all nurses agree with mutual recognition as the solution for interstate practice. Most of the opposition seems to stem from concern about the inequality of standards for nurse practitioner practice from one state to another. Basic nurse education is very standardized across states, but because of the widely varied requirements for practice for nurse practitioners, these nurses were excluded from the current compact being implemented.

Congress and telehealth advocates have recognized a need to eliminate interstate licensure barriers, nursing must also work to eliminate these barriers. Nursing has an opportunity to move forward and become a role model for other health care providers in the issue of interstate practice. The mutual recognition model is designed to eliminate the cost of multiple licenses and to clarify jurisdiction for interstate practice. The ANA 1999 House of Delegates agreed to recognize mutual recognition as one of the approaches for regulating interstate/multistate practice. Hopefully, nursing will accept the challenges of interstate practice and move forward to try to solve the issue, rather than sitting back and allowing others to develop a structure that would hinder individual nurses from participating in telehealth practice.

Security of Information

For many years, the informatics community has expressed concern about the lack of adequate regulations to secure patient records. Because telehealth technologies electronically transmit patient information over wide geographic areas, concerns about the security of identifiable health information have intensified. The Health Insurance Portability and Accountability Act (HIPAA) of 1996 mandates that standard regulations regarding security of patient information be adopted.

Security standards will apply to health plans, health care clearinghouses, and health care providers who transmit health information electronically. Protection will be required when information becomes electronic. Information becomes electronic either when it is sent electronically as a transaction or by being maintained in a computer system. Information is covered under the regulations if it has any components that could identify a subject.

Security regulations under HIPAA will preempt state laws that may be in conflict with the regulatory requirements and that provide less stringent protection. Failure to comply with the regulations could result in monetary penalties. According to these regulations, wrongful disclosures of protected health information could evoke criminal penalties (DHHS, 1999). Needless to say, once they are enacted the HIPAA security regulations will have tremendous impact on how clinical data is handled by nurses, physicians, and other providers during and after a telehealth event.

Competence

As stated earlier, some would like to see telehealth practice for nurses become a specialty practice, complete with certification. Again the question is what would be the domain of interest. Since the purpose of telehealth practice is to increase access to quality health care, the focus should remain on clinical care. During telehealth encounters, nurses use their clinical knowledge and skills to interact with patients and/or to present them to consulting practitioners. Telehealth technologies simply enable that process to occur at a distance.

It is worrisome that some nurses are pushing for certification in telehealth. This author believes that requiring nurses to be certified in telehealth would severely limit the availability of health care providers in rural and frontier areas that could participate in telehealth events. As a result, patients could be denied access to quality care. And nurses could be unnecessarily denied opportunities to practice using the tools of telehealth technology. Requiring certification for nurses using telehealth technologies will also have implications for reimbursement. If certification is required, it is probable that within a short time reimbursement will be denied unless the provider meets that requirement. Such action could hinder the expansion of telehealth programs to underserved populations that desperately need these services.

There is no doubt that interacting with patients electronically changes communication patterns. But interacting with patients that have endotracheal tubes or are visually challenged also changes communication patterns. One of nursing's strengths is being able to adapt clinical practice to different types of environments encountered while delivering care. This includes the environment of telehealth.

In 1998, the ANA convened a panel of nursing organization representatives to identify needed competencies for nurses engaged in telehealth practice. There was much discussion about the issue of whether telehealth practice is a specialty, but the group discounted telehealth as a specialty and agreed that clinical practice standards should guide telehealth practice. This conclusion is consistent with the first principle listed in the core principles of a telehealth document (ANA, 1999). That document resulted from an earlier collaborative project between the Joint Working Group on Telemedicine, a Federal interagency group that focuses on telehealth, and the ANA.

Eleven competencies were identified that address the broad variety of settings where nurses might use telehealth technologies. The eleven proposed competencies are:

- Adapts nursing practice to integrate telehealth,
- Establishes a therapeutic relationship with the patient,
- Assesses appropriate communication and adjusts techniques as needed,
- Assesses appropriateness of telehealth technologies in specific situations,
- Determines whether client needs can be met with telehealth technologies,
- Demonstrates competent knowledge and skill is using technologies, Ensures privacy, confidentiality, informed consent, and security, Demonstrates skill in performing a consultation,
- Modifies practice according to results of telehealth performance improvement activities, and
- Documents the telehealth event (ANA Invitational Meeting, March 30–31, 1998).

Cost of Telehealth

In today's health care environment, any treatment modality, even those involving technology, should be evaluated in terms of the cost. Cost information about telehealth projects is not readily available.

The ORHP attempted to determine the costs of patient encounters using telemedicine. However, not all non-Federal rural hospitals in the 1997 study reported the costs of their telemedicine projects. Those reporting start up costs most frequently indicated spending $100,000 to $500,000 for telemedicine equipment. New programs (less than one year) most commonly spent $50 to $200 for transmission costs per session. More established programs spent less than $50 per session for transmission. The number of telemedicine events was determined and a median unit cost per session calculated (ORHP, 1997). The results show a cost of between $500 and $1000 per session, depending on whether the site is a spoke or hub site respectively.

Although the costs seem high for each telehealth session and the need for empirical telemedicine research is widely recognized, one has to examine additional variables when determining the true costs of telehealth. Many patients would be denied earlier and less costly care if providers did not have access to services delivered through telehealth. For example, Rendina and Carrasco (1999) show that neonates received earlier treatment for cardiac disorders by telemedicine transmission of echocardiograms, thereby preventing more severe complications of their disease associated with delay of treatment. In addition, transportation rates and the length of stay in newborn intensive care units were significantly reduced (Rendina & Carrasco, 1999). Brunicardi (1998) demonstrated savings when a volume of patients was treated within Ohio's prison system rather than transporting them. Factors such as this must be considered when calculating the costs of telehealth.

Other factors are not as easily measured. How do you determine cost savings associated with the alleviation of emotional distress? A telepathology event could allow a woman in a small rural hospital to receive an immediate diagnosis of non-malignant breast mass rather than having to wait several days for the specimen to be sent to a larger health care facility for evaluation.

The purpose of telehealth is to increase access to care. As access is increased, those needing care might use additional services. Initially/telehealth may seem to increase health care costs for payers, but if it is also used to provide preventive services, particularly to the underserved populations, telehealth may save health care dollars.

Meantime, the cost of equipment for delivering telehealth care may need to be considered part of the cost of doing business, and not an expense that must show an absolute return on investment (ROI). For many years, the informatics community tried unsuccessfully to demonstrate an ROI for information systems. Once information became valued as a business commodity, such efforts were in large part abandoned.

This author suggests a similar view for telehealth technologies. As equipment becomes more standardized and less proprietary, costs for starting telehealth programs should be reduced. Evidence-based practice is needed for telehealth. Efforts should be focused on determining best practices for using telehealth rather than on classic cost/benefit analysis for using telehealth technologies. Hopefully, nursing will position itself to be part of telehealth evaluation efforts, especially as it relates to those areas of telehealth that are well-served by nurses.

TELEHEALTH AND INFORMATICS

It is interesting that separate telehealth and informatics conferences have been held internationally, nationally, and locally for several years. Consequently, attendees discuss similar issues without benefit of sharing information about potential solutions. It seems more logical to consider telehealth technology systems as a type of information system that uses primarily imaging for exchanging information. Bringing the audiences together would facilitate the development of solutions for problems such as equipment interface standards, security of information, archiving of information, and interdisciplinary language requirements for documentation of telehealth events.

There is evidence that the two interest areas are coming together. For example, the American Medical Informatics Association has recently established a telehealth special interest group. In another example, the University of California, Davis has been recognized for forging a formal relationship between telemedicine and informatics in their institution (Dakins & Kincade, 1999).

INCREASING TELEHEALTH IN NURSING

Nursing involvement in telehealth has resulted in some very exciting programs. Lewis, McCann, Hidalgo, & Gorman (1997) used store-

and-forward telehealth technologies to transmit images of vascular wounds to a vascular nurse clinician in a regional medical center. Goldsmith and Safran (1999) used the web to instruct ambulatory patients about their surgery and significantly reduce postoperative pain. There are other examples of nurses using telehealth to provide clinical care, but more nurses need to demonstrate how the use of telehealth technologies can positively impact clients in their homes and in underserved areas. To successfully apply for available telehealth Federal funding, nurses should consider collaborating with other health care entities and/or disciplines as needed to establish comprehensive telehealth programs. There are several agencies within the Federal government that fund telehealth projects. Telehealth projects listed in the Federal Telemedicine Directory (HRSA, 1998) were funded by eight different government agencies. Possible government funding sources are listed in Table 12.1.

SUMMARY

The new millennium is here, but the challenge to deliver quality and cost effective care to all Americans remains a priority. Nursing has an opportunity to become a leader in telehealth practice. Nursing should focus on those who are receiving no health care and populations in underserved areas; deliver care to the elderly in their homes; collaborate with other health care providers to identify telehealth best practice models of care; and work to eliminate barriers for expanding the use of telehealth technologies.

TABLE 12.1 Federal Telehealth Funding Agencies

Department	Agency	Program	Internet address
Agriculture	Rural Utilities Service	Distance learning and Telemedicine Program	www.usda.gov/rus/dlt/dlml.htm
Appalachian Regional Commission		Telecommunications	www.arc.gov
Commerce	National Telecommunications and Information Administration	Office of Telecommunications and Information Applications	www.ntia.doc.gov/otia home/otiahome.html
Defense			www.defenselink.mil
Education		Prepare, teachers to use technology	www.ed.gov
Health and Human Services	Agency for Healthcare Research and Quality		www.ahrq..gov
Health and Human Services	Health Care Financial Administration	Special projects	www.hcfa.gov
Health and Human Services	Indian Health Service		www.ihs.gov

TABLE 12.1 *(continued)*

Department	Agency	Program	Internet address
Health and Human Services	Health Resources and Services Administration	Office of Rural Health Policy	www.nal.usda.gov/orhp
Health and Human Services	Health Resources and Services Administration	Office for the Advancement of Telehealth	http://telehealth.hrsa.gov
Health and Human Services	National Institutes of Health	National Library of Medicine	www.nlm.nih.gov
National Aeronautics and Space Administration			www.nasa.gov
National Science Foundation			www.nsf.gov
Veterans Affairs			www.va.gov

REFERENCES

American Nurses Association (1997). *Status report on telenursing and telehealth.* Washington, DC: American Nurses Association.

American Nurses Association (1999). *Core principles on telehealth.* Washington, DC: American Nurses Publishing.

Brunicaradi, B. O. (1998). Financial analysis of savings from telemedicine in Ohio's prison system. *Telemedicine Journal, 4*(1), 49–54.

Chaffee, M. (1999). A telehealth odyssey. *American Journal of Nursina, 99*(7), 27–30.

Conrad, K. (1977). Introduction. *North Dakota Law Review, 73*(1), 1–6.

Dakins, D. R. (1997). Market targets 1997. *Telemedicine and Telehealth Networks, 3*(3), 25–29

Dakins, D. R. (1999). Increased investment and incremental expansion fuels optimism. *Telehealth Magazine, 5*(3), 28–31.

Dakins, D. R., & Kincade, K. (1998). The envelope, please: Top 10 telemedicine programs for 1998. *Telehealth Macazine, 4*(7), 32–33, 35, 37, 40–41, 43, 45, 47–48.

Dansky, K. H., Bowles, K. H., & Palmer, L. (1999). How telehomecare affects patients. *Caring, August 1999,* 10–14

Department of Health and Humari services (1999). Proposed standards for privacy of individually identifiable health information. Available [on-line]: *http://aspe.hhs.gov/adminsimp/pvcsumm.htm.*

Goldsmith, D. M., & Safran, C. (1999). Using the web to reduce postoperative pain following ambulatory surgery. In N. M. Lorenzi (Ed.), *Journal of the American Medical Informatics Association: Proceedings of AMIA '98 Annual Symposium, November 6–10, 1999* (pp. 380–384). Philadelphia: Hanley & Belfus.

Health Resources and Services Administration (1997). *Federal Telemedicine Directory, 1997.* Washington, DC: Department of Health and Human Services.

Health Resources and Services Administration (1998). *Federal Telemedicine Directorv, 1998.* Washington, DC: Department of Health and Human Services.

Hutcherson, C., & Williamson, S. H. (1999). Nursing regulation for the new millennium: The mutual recognition model. *Online Journal of Issues in Nursing.* May 31, 1999. [On-Line] Available: *http://www.nursingworld.org/ojin/topic9/topic9_2.htm.*

Institute of Medicine (1996). *Telemedicine: A guide to assessing telecom-*

munications in health care. Washington, DC: National Academy Press.

Kincade, K. (1999). "Hall of Fame" members share secrets of success. *Telehealth Maaazine, 5*(4), 30–33.

Levy, B. (1999, October). Regulating the practice of medicine across state lines. Paper presented at the conference for the Center for Telehealth Law, Washington, DC.

Lewis, P., McCann, R., & Gorman, M. (1997). Use of store and forward technology for vascular nursing teleconsultation service. *Journal of Vascular Nursing, 15*(4), 116–123.

National Council of State Boards of Nursing (1996). Telenursing: The regulatory implications for multistate regulation. [On-Line] Available: *www.ncsbn.org/files/publications/issues/vol173/telenurs173.asp.*

Office of Rural Health Policy (1997). *Exploratory evaluation of rural applications of telemedicine.* Rockville, MD: Health Resources and Services Administration, DHHS.

PEW Health Professions Commission (1998). *Strengthening consumer protection: Priorities for health care workforce regulation.* San Francisco: University of California. The Center for the Health Professions.

Rendina, M. C., & Carrasco, N. (1999). Beyond feasibility: Neonatal telecardiology shows cost benefits. *Telehealth Magazine, 5*(3), 24–27, 37.

Sharp, N. (1998). Teleconsultation: The death of distance. *The Nurse Practitioner, 23*(10), 84, 87–88

Telehealth Magazine (1998). Online survey results offer telemedicine practice insights. *Telehealth Magazine, 4*(6), 10–11.

Tracey, J. (1999, October). Removing regulatory barriers: A telemedicine panel. Panel presentation at the conference of the Center for Telemedicine Law, Washington, DC.

Waters. R. J. (1999, October). Practicing beyond borders: Health professional licensure in the new millennium. Paper presented at the conference of the Center for Telehealth Law, Washington, DC.

13

Nursing Informatics In the Home Health Care Environment
Catherine O. Mallard

Home health care is reinventing itself. Changes in regulations and reimbursement are forcing certified home health care agencies to redefine how they conduct business (St. Pierre, 1999). For decades, the federal government through its Medicare program has been the largest payer source for home care services. Starting in 1998, the Health Care Financing Administration (HCFA) issued changes in regulations that brought decreased reimbursement with the introduction of the interim payment system (IPS), additional data collection requirements (Dombi & St. Pierre, 1999), and in June 2000, the final regulations for a prospective payment system (PPS) were published and are effective as of October 2000.

This is not unlike what took place in the hospital industry when Medicare replaced fee-for-service reimbursement with the Diagnoses Related Groups (DRG) payment model. PPS for homecare uses a classification system consisting of 80 Home Health Resource Group (HHRG), also called HRGs, which will be the basis of payment for each 80-day episode. Home care agencies are maintaining their existence by diversifying services and expanding their patient population while competing with other agencies locked in the same struggle. Agencies are streamlining their business processes, offering new services, developing market awareness, and trying to better manage the cost and quality of care.

Information technology is essential in the new environment to access, integrate, and interchange data across networks from referrers to vendors, physicians, network providers, hospitals, and government agencies. It presents new ways of doing business—point of service systems, website access, and telehealth applications. Additionally, information systems capture vital information for analysis of payer sources, service volume, utilization, patient data, and the outcomes of care.

REGULATORY ENVIRONMENT

Home health services are covered under Part A and B of the Medicare Program. Certified home health agencies (CHHA) must meet the Conditions of Participation (COP) in the Medicare Program as stipulated by HCFA. These conditions stipulate documentation guidelines, and specify the level and type of services covered and the time frames required for getting signed physician orders. Medicare recipients must meet certain eligibility requirements to receive home health care. They must be homebound, require the provision of skilled services (nursing and/or rehabilitation therapy), and services must be needed on an interim basis only, not continuously.

CHHAs must maintain a plan of care or medical plan of treatment for all their patients. The physician's plan of care specifies the patient's functional status, activities permitted, prognosis for rehabilitation, medications, visit frequency, and duration for each service, discipline specific treatments, medical goals, and discharge plan. Services include nursing, physical therapy, occupational therapy, speech therapy, and paraprofessional (home health aide). The plan of care is commonly referred to as the HCFA 485 (the number on the HCFA form). It is created by the agency and sent to the patient's primary physician for signature. The plan of care must be reviewed and signed by a physician to recertify patient care for any additional 60-day period. CHHAs must follow these regulations for all patients admitted to the agency regardless of payer source to meet the COP.

Reimbursement

Until 1998, Medicare reimbursement for home health services was retrospective and paid on a fee-for-service basis. Agencies billed for the number of professional and paraprofessional visits provided. In 1998, HCFA enacted the Interim Payment System (IPS) in order to reduce Medicare spending specified by the Balanced Budget Act of

1997 (Berke, 1998), and to begin the transition to a prospective payment system. IPS reduced reimbursement for home health agencies based on a formula using each agency's 1995 cost reports. The effects were dramatic. At its 1999 annual convention, the National Association for Home Care (NAHC) reported that close to 2,500 agencies closed as a result. Agencies that survived adapted their practices to the new environment. The formula of more visits equals more revenue was reversed under IPS to less visits equals more revenue. New strategies had to be found to care for patients with chronic conditions such as diabetes, congestive heart failure, and venous stasis ulcers without abandoning those in need of services (Dombi & St. Pierre, 1999).

CHHAs were further pressed in 1998 when Medicare revised its COP to require a standardized national assessment tool called OASIS (*O*utcomes *AS*sessment *I*nformation *S*et) be integrated into an agency's assessment. The OASIS assessment is a data set of 100+ questions designed and tested by the University of Colorado (Shaughnessy, Crisler, Schlenker, Arnold, Kramer et al, 1994). The purpose of the OASIS is to provide a standardized assessment to evaluate functional and cognitive outcomes for the purpose of clinical outcome based quality improvement. Importantly, the OASIS is also the basis for the beneficiary's case-mix that has three components: clinical, functional, and service utilization. The PPS case-mix classification system uses select data elements from the OASIS assessment to reflect different patient conditions.

The regulations state that OASIS assessments must be completed for all nonmaternity patients over 18 years of age. These assessments are done at regular intervals coinciding with the medical plan of treatment: at the start of care (admission), at intervals of every 60 days (recertification), at the time of hospitalization, and at discharge from the certified agency. The guidelines released by HCFA are explicit and rigid as to time frames, explanation of questions and requirements for electronic submission of data (Mikos & Koch, 1999).

In October of 1999, HCFA published the proposed rule for implementation of the prospective payment system (PPS). This was followed by the PPS final regulation in June of 2000. PPS will alter the payment methodology from the current retrospective reasonable cost-based system to one that will reimburse-home health agencies based on a 60-day episode of care (HCFA, 1999). A significant element in the PPS rate structure is the case mix adjuster. The rule specifies 80 Home Health Resource Groups (HHRG) to which a patient may be assigned. Three dimensions determine a patient's classification: clinical, functional, and service utilization. A patient is classified in these categories based on a numeric value associated with the score on certain OASIS questions. PPS scheduled for implementation in October 2000. Although PPS corrects the payment inequities of IPS with the establishment of a national 60-day episode payment that is adjusted for case-mix and geographical wage levels, the PPS requirements potentially staggering to the industry (McSpedon, 1999; St. Pierre, 1999). At the least, agencies will need to convert financial and information systems to accommodate new billing and accounting needs. This puts home health care in the midst of a turbulent transition.

STATE OF INFORMATION SYSTEMS

In 1999, there were 8,734 Medicare certified home health care agencies in the United States (National Association for Home Care, May 1999 statistics, reported by telephone). The typical agency has 486 admissions and 30,000 visits/yr. and a staff of 50 and a small profit margin. The decision to purchase a clinical information system is a large financial commitment. Up to the present, the chief demand in home care has been for financial systems. Similar to other businesses, home health care is reliant on computers to generate bills and track receivables.

In most instances, the clinical data maintained electronically has been limited to services specified on the medical treatment order/plan of care, the HCFA 485. The rest of the medical record, assessments, clinical progress notes, and paraprofessional care is maintained manually. Home care has been slow to implement clinical information systems, but that must change in a PPS environment. Agencies are investigating the purchase of point-of-care systems and transitioning from manual systems.

The need to move toward a point-of-care system has been driven by several factors. With Medicare reimbursement diminished, home health care has looked to contract with other payers. Managed care has been a growing source of revenue. A home care agency has to furnish various data on managed care clients in order to acquire that business. Managed care companies expect agency report cards with data on number of admissions, number of visits, type of services provided, sorted by diagnoses, and even by zip code. If possible, payers would like to be furnished with outcome data (Geraci, 1997). Contractors, payers, and physicians expect to have full access to relevant patient data.

The implementation of PPS will demand that agencies scrupulously manage the patient's 60-day episode of care. The agency must monitor its care practices in relation to utilization and have the ability to analyze and predict case-mix based on HHRG scores from the OASIS. Outcome data will be critical for determining cost effectiveness and efficiency of care management. None of this is possible without information technology.

Nursing Data and Information in System Development

Nurses furnish the majority of service in home care. Given this fact it follows that the available software has been developed primarily for nursing documentation. The structure of the documentation is based on what is most commonly documented on paper progress notes. In some instances it is a lexicon of words and phrases that the user can string together into sentence structures. In other cases, the nursing actions are statements constructed in sequence based on nursing practice, that is, the actions a nurse would document when treating a patient with a right atrial catheter.

Two nurses who have made important contributions to nursing informatics within the home health care field are Dr. Virginia K. Saba who authored the Home Health Care Classification (HHCC) and Karen Martin who was the lead developer of the Omaha System.

The Home Health Care Classification is a standardized nomenclature designed specifically for a computer-based home health care system (Saba, 1997). There are 20 nursing care components, for example, cardiac, coping, and nutritional that comprises the nursing framework. In addition the system links to nursing diagnoses and nursing interventions. Each nursing diagnosis requires Outcome Identification evaluated at discharge. The three qualifiers are: Improved, Stabilized, or Deteriorated. These are the same descriptors used in the measurement of outcomes for the OASIS.

The Omaha System came out of research conducted at the VNA of Omaha. It has three schema: Problem Classification; Intervention, and Problem Rating Scale for Outcomes (Martin, & Scheet, 1992). Together they present the clinician with a interdisciplinary tool to organize and interpret information. It has been used across health care settings, including community health and long-term care.

Computers In Home Health Care

In the home health care milieu, mobile computing is the only technology solution. Home care professionals are mobile workers whose workplace extends beyond the office. Care is given in patients' homes and documentation is done wherever and whenever it's convenient— which may be in the patient's home, the car, or the clinician's home. The organization must equip each field staff member with a mobile computer (i.e., laptop, notebook, pen-based or handheld device) with the capability for remote dial-up or wireless communication in order to automate the clinical record (Mallard & Mitchell, 1998).

A home care agency has to determine the feasibility of funding this effort and conduct a cost benefit analysis. The return on investment cannot be measured in strictly financial terms (Mead, 1995).

Some of the benefits of an automated system allow an agency to streamline business operations and reduce back office processing, and to increase productivity by reducing travel time to and from the office. Agencies that invest in automated clinical systems have the ability to collect and report relevant clinical care and outcome data to payers. As stated previously, this is increasingly important in today's health care market. Putting computers in the hands of the field staff provides access to the most up-to-date patient information, provides a tool to support clinical decision making and care delivery, provides a standard for documentation, automates entry of physician's orders, and incorporates practice and regulatory guidelines (Mallard & Mitchell, 1998; Mead, 1995). These benefits, however, are difficult to measure. The agency has to weigh them against the cost and make a decision that is sound for the organization. "There are three popular techniques to assess economic feasibility, also called *cost-effectiveness*: payback analysis, return on investment, and net present value." (Whitten & Bentley, 1998, p. 652).

SYSTEM SELECTION

The next phase is system selection. The major activities include researching the system technology available in the marketplace, defining the business and technology requirements, preparing a request for proposal (RFP), reviewing vendor proposals, and recommending the system that best meets the business requirements (Whitten & Bentley, 1998). This is a major undertaking and should not be underestimated. In home care, the two major stakeholders are nursing and information systems. Nursing represents the majority of the clinical system user group and must be a strong presence throughout the procurement phase. It is not uncommon, however, for the decision to rest with the information systems department (I.S.). I.S. has the background and experience with computer technology. It is critical that nursing educate itself about the available technology and not relinquish its authority in the decision-making process.

A first step is to assemble a steering committee and/or project team with interdepartmental representation. The organizational management of the project can take many forms depending on the size of the organization. One option is to have a steering committee with administrative heads from nursing, operations, finance, and information systems departments. The role of this committee would be to review and finalize decisions related to equipment purchases, system selection, budget, project plans, etc. A project team with representation from middle management would also be assembled. The members of this group manage the day-to-day project tasks and report periodically to the steering committee. As the main user, nursing needs to take ownership of the project. In this scenario, the nursing director chairs the executive committee, and a member of the information systems staff serves as project director. This allows for a balance of power between the two primary departments involved. However, it is more important that whoever heads the project has the leadership characteristics needed for success. These include understanding the big picture, articulating a coherent vision for the future, establishing clear goals, using appropriate leadership styles based on the situation, and learning from both successes and failures. (Lorenzi, Riley, Ball, & Douglas, 1995).

As the person with the most in-depth knowledge about the clinical requirements, the nursing representative on the project team must be on equal footing with the staff from other departments. Computer systems are unfamiliar territory for most clinicians—the technical aspects, even the language, are bewildering. The clinical representative needs to be familiar with the state of the agency's computer systems and future data requirements—both internal and external to the organization. Without this background, the clinical representative will have difficulty evaluating the available software and technology options.

The people assigned to the project team must be able to devote the time required to accomplish the task and be prepared to continue on the project team until its conclusion. The knowledge gained from the initial phases will help the team make informed decisions.

The most pressing task facing the project team is defining what the organization needs and wants from the new system. This will entail developing specifications that outline the business and clinical requirements of the system, and a broad description of the data inputs and outputs (Whitten & Bentley, 1998). Having determined the prerequisites of the system, the team can determine whether it is best to build or to buy a system. Few home care agencies have the clinical and technology resources to build a system in-house. Given the magnitude of the project, the team may issue a request for proposal (RFP) using the system specifications they have developed. As part of the RFP process, the team establishes the selection criteria by which it will evaluate the vendor proposals.

The majority of software vendors with home care systems offer integrated financial and clinical components. One consideration that has considerable influence on the selection of a clinical system is its compatibility with the financial system. If the systems are being purchased together it is important that the clinical and the financial sides of the system be given equal thought as to functionality and user friendliness (Table 13.1: Vendor Issues).

The team should keep in mind that vendors want to sell their product. They are going to present their software in the most favorable of terms. The other warning is what you see may not be what you get. Software is constantly being upgraded. The product demonstrated at trade shows is often the latest development prototype with all the bells and whistles to entice the customer. The team should ascertain if what they are seeing is the production version or a future

TABLE 13.1 Vendor Issues

A few questions to consider when examining available products include:

1. Does it support the agency's strategic initiatives?
2. Does the software address defined information needs?
3. Does it support clinical decision making and care delivery?
4. Is it user friendly?
5. Is it compatible with existing applications?
6. What are the hardware requirements?
7. What support does the vendor provide to users?

release. A ". . . major issue is *vendor misinformation. A* practical rule is that the newer the technology, the more inflated and/or misleading the vendor claims will be" (Lorenzi et al., 1995, p. 42.). The sales people do not have all the technical information, and a technical expert rarely attends an initial demonstration. The project team should meet with a technical expert during the selection phase.

The vendor will supply references and assist the team to arrange site visits to organizations where the system is fully implemented and clinicians are using the software in the field. The nursing team member participates on the visit. It is an opportunity to meet with managers and field staff, to learn the pros and cons of the software, and to see it in operation. A useful approach for these meetings is to ask about a specific process, that is, Could you explain how changes in the plan of care are done and is there automated tracking of the physician's order? This will provide an inside view on a critical home care process that crosses clinical and financial lines. With a mobile workforce, ease of use is essential and easily ascertained by accompanying a clinician in the field. "User friendly" may be a hackneyed phrase, but it has to be kept in mind when reviewing software products. While on the site visit, it is a good idea to establish a nursing contact at the site to call with follow-up questions.

Moving Forward

The time frame from selection of a clinical system to implementation can range anywhere from 12 months to over 2 years. There are several factors that influence this, such as, the size of the agency, the complexity of the communication infrastructure, the hardware selection and purchase, the resources assigned to the implementation, and the amount of customization. For purposes of this discussion, the focus will be on resources and customization.

Devoting adequate resources is most essential to the project's success. The original project team may assume responsibility for implementation, or it may be reorganized around this next phase. As stated previously, the project director is generally a member of I.S. The person selected should have experience managing a project and be familiar with the current systems and documentation standards. The project director coordinates and oversees the technology and clinical aspects of the project, and keeps the steering or executive committee apprised of the team's progress (Lorenzi et al., 1995).

The nurse serving on the project team may take on the responsibilities of a project manager. Depending on the organization, the project manager may retain a position in nursing with a dotted line to the project director or report directly to I.S. Regardless, the project manager is liaison between the nursing department and the vendor on clinical matters, plans and oversees the training and implementation, and works directly with the system analyst. The system analyst directs the data design of the clinical system based on the organizational requirements and the product's functionality, and helps troubleshoot problems once the system is implemented (Whitten & Bentley, 1998). Ideally, this person should have a background in nursing given that in home care the clinical aspects are integrated with the functionality of the financial systems and business processes.

The system analyst will devote a large amount of time to fact-finding, a process by which he/she will learn about the vocabulary, constraints, requirements, and priorities of the business and of the system (Whitten & Bentley,1998). For instance, for an agency to bill for services it must have signed physician orders. When the nurse enters into the system a verbal order from the physician to change a patient's visit frequency, the system must track the order to ensure that it was sent to the physician and received back signed. The system analyst will need to understand how this is done currently in the organization, if the automated system supports this business activity, and the required data inputs and outputs.

Design Phase

Software does not exist that can satisfy every user. It is a rare organization that buys a product and uses it "as is" (Whitten & Bentley, 1998). Once the contract is signed, the organization will begin the process of customizing the software. During this phase, the system analyst will ensure that the software solution meets the business and clinical requirements as defined. All software can be customized—to an extent. The core functionality, the functions a user can perform when using the software, usually cannot be modified. Presumably, the product was selected because it was judged as the overall best. Other areas that are generally off limits for customization are the data structures. "Data structures are specific arrangements of data attributes [the smallest piece of data that has meaning to end-users and business] that define the organization of a singe instance of a data flow" (Whitten & Bentley, 1998, p. 230). An example of a data structure is an address that contains these data attributes: street address, city, state, and zip code.

The vendor will outline the areas where agency specific data is required, such as payer codes, vendor names, and physician information. The vendor will build items such as discharge reasons, which are organization-specific, into a "user-defined" table as part of the application development for the agency.

The area most open for customization is the content. Deciding what content to customize and then developing the content is a daunting task. A clinical documentation system will include content, such as predetermined assessments and clinical documentation structures. Generally, vendors will allow an amount of customization. The ability to modify the content depends on the functionality built into the application. The system analyst has the necessary knowledge to lead the data design (Whitten & Bentley, 1998). A representative group of users, clinical field staff and managers, reviews the clinical data available with the system and makes recommendations. The recommended content changes are ranked in priority starting with essentials. Customizing software outside of the user defined tables can be very costly and add weeks, if not months, to a project. The system analyst ascertains that the suggested changes are feasible before submitting them, for example, the request for an assessment tool that produces a patient-specific score is not realistic if the assessment module does not have the ability to do calculations. The group should also be asked to answer the following questions. Can the nurses use the system as is? Can the modifications or enhancements be delivered in phases once the system is implemented? Are the modifications or enhancements within the functionality of the application? If the answers are yes, data design can go on simultaneous with the implementation. If no, then the importance of the modifications and/or enhancements has to be weighed against the cost and the impact on the implementation schedule.

Once the list is finalized, the project director contacts the vendor for an estimate of the time and the cost before approving the changes. If the delivery of the modifications will delay the project or result in cost overruns, the steering or executive committee should be apprised and decide the issue.

Work Flow

The implementation of an automated system in any environment is a major change. It is essential that the participants understand what will change as the organization converts from its old systems to a new system. If a business process redesign was conducted at the beginning of the selection phase, the organization will have identified how the introduction of the new system will change the current business and clinical processes (Whitten & Bentley, 1998). It will be important to actually involve people in learning how their jobs will be different. (Lorenzi et al., 1995).

A work flow analysis is useful in examining the current work processes in light of the new system's known functionality—what the user can do on the system and how the data flows. Although the requirements were defined as part of the selection phase, the system purchased may not meet all requirements. The work flow will ascertain how data is processed, for example, how the system processes a change in payer; where are the potential fail points, what are the consequences if there is a communication failure, etc.

In home care, the workflow starts with the referral of the patient to the agency. One of the first questions is how are referrals tracked now, and how will the system handle this function? Next, how does the system handle patient assignment to a nurse? What information is given to the nurse at the time of referral now—what information will be on the computer, can the nurse retrieve the information in the field? Will the nurse dial in remotely from the field? How does the manager know the nurse received the information? What is documented on the initial visit—is this done on the computer? A sample workflow (Table 13.2: Sample Work Flow) is provided to illustrate an agency's work flow related to the process 60-day recertifications.

TABLE 13.2 Sample Work Flow

CLINICIAN:
- Receives notice via pen-based computer 10 days in advance of when physician authorization is due for recertification of service
- Between days 56 to 60 of the certification period, completes the 60-day OASIS comprehensive assessment and recertification
- System ensures completeness of required fields, that is, visit frequency and duration
- Designates physician/clinic to receive Recertification forms
- Signs Recertification on-line with PIN
- Transmits data collected via modem

SUPERVISOR
- Reviews Recertification On-line Worklist on a daily basis. Selects patient and accesses Recertification Plan of Care on-line for review. Returns to worklist to approve and release Recertification for printing at local printer.

CLERK:
- Sends (faxes or mails) Recertification form and 60-day summary to physician/clinic for signature and return to agency.

SUPERVISOR:
- Reviews and initials signed Recertification when received back at the agency office.
- Enters into system any changes made by the physician to the Recertification Plan of Care. Informs clinician of changes.
- Forwards to Clerk for filing.

CLERK:
- Enters into Plan of Care tracking system that Recertification Form was signed and received. Follows current procedure regarding filing into Medical Record.

The work flow was developed by the Visiting Nurse Service of New York as part of the implementation of its clinical system.

Going through this analysis and answering these questions and innumerable others is an essential activity. The result will furnish the organization with an indispensable document that is revisited as the project progresses and serves as a training tool during implementation.

I.S. staff participates in the work flow discussions or is available to advise the group. They have critical information related to the design of the communications infrastructure, a vital area in home health care. The work flow is influenced by whether or not the clinician has remote dial-in capability, and what information is updated during the communication session. Relevant information provided by the I.S. department includes a description of what data is transmitted to the clinician and when; how updates to the patient data are handled—in real time or by batch; what happens when two nurses are assigned to one patient; what can be printed from the system; what management reports can be generated; and how the system ensures confidentiality of patient data.

The work flow analysis can result in recommendations to modify the system design or functionality. Only those functional changes that are deemed critical to the business should be submitted.

The work flow analysis is an optimal time to look at how the introduction of an automated system changes existing policies and to identify where new policies will need to be developed. For example, the Clinical Practice Manual has to reflect how a discharge is performed electronically as compared to a paper discharge. A policy for use of an electronic signature by the clinician needs to be written, as well as how the system maintains confidentiality of patient information. The vendor may provide an agency with this information written in terms that meet regulatory requirements, but it is the agency's responsibility to insure that HCFA regulations are met.

IMPLEMENTATION

An important aspect of implementation is to prepare a conversion plan to ensure a smooth transition to the new system (Whitten & Bentley, 1998). This includes conducting system tests, installing databases, and loading agency specific data, such as lists of payers, physician information, vendors, and information on active patients. The timing as to when the system goes into production is dependent on the completion of this work .

It is customary to run a pilot with a new system. The pilot involves a limited number of staff and is of sufficient length to test the performance of all system applications to see that they are working properly under all conditions and business scenarios. In home care, a suggested time frame for the pilot is 90 days. This allows the monitoring of the system through the recertification process, a critical activity in home care. During the pilot, the agency runs parallel systems—meaning keeping the manual or current systems in place while implementing the new automated system. This is stipulated as part of the conversion plan. The pilot design details the monitoring of critical data, that is, data accuracy, corroboration that data are hitting the correct fields in the system, and ensuring that data is being transmitted accurately and completely. Problems stemming from user error and system bugs will occur. That is the purpose of the pilot. It is what makes it worthwhile.

During the pilot, the information systems department monitors system performance and communications. This includes measuring how long it takes data to be transmitted to and from the nurse's computer, the system's ability to handle multiple nurses communicating simultaneously, and tracking reported communication problems. This will be important information in the evaluation phase.

The pilot is also a test of the vendor's support capability. Nothing else simulates going live with the system in the real environment. The problems will vary in nature and criticality. The vendor may monitor the system on site or remotely. Either way, it is important to gather adequate data to analyze the problem and determine how best to apply a remedy. With a purchased system, it is possible to learn what other agencies experienced during implementation, and the quality of the vendor's response.

Training

Training is fundamental to a successful implementation—regardless of the computer application. Home care presents a unique challenge. Clinical staff uses the system in the field; they are mobile workers. They can't ask the person next to them what to do when they have a problem. Training has to be organized to make them independent users with the ability to manage equipment as well as successfully use the application. Vendors may offer an established training program including a train-the-trainer programs so that agency staff can deliver the training. Vendors often work with buyers to customize the training as needed. See Table 13.3: Training Issues.

The training plan must suit the needs of the agency. Availability of trainers and nurses is an important issue that needs to be dealt with at the start. Taking nurses out of the field for days of training is a hardship for many agencies. One strategy is to organize the training into half-day sessions to accommodate operations. Whatever schedule is decided, it is important that operations agree to the schedule and support attendance. The sooner schedules can be delivered to the clinical managers, the better they can arrange staff coverage.

Hands-on training is the only approach to use when teaching a computer application. The class follows the training exercise and performs the functions along with the instructor. Surveys and pre-tests are two ways to determine how much time to spend on computer basics.

One objective of training is to ensure that users are competent in using the application. Small classes facilitate training and allow instructors to assist users who have difficulty and to identify users who need additional training. Homework assignments allow users to independently access and enter data on the system. The assignment can

TABLE 13.3 Basic Training curriculum might include:

- Care and maintenance of the equipment,
- Introduction to Windows Conventions, that is, minimizing and closing programs
- Communication, including e-mail, if available
- How to access patient information
- How to update demographics and financial information
- How to maintain the plan of care
- How to enter a visit
- How to perform an assessment, including OASIS

be scored as an objective measure of user competency. It demonstrates their ability to navigate the application, to locate information within the application, and to correctly enter information, and suggests to them areas where they need help. It is useful for the instructors to develop course evaluations for the students to rate the training experience. If problems are identified, the training is revised before further training is held. This is useful data for the evaluation.

Providing support once users go live on the system is a must. Nothing ever goes as planned. Problems are inevitable and it is best to be prepared. The primary goal is to ensure that help is available to the clinical staff when they need it. Having the trainers in the field is ideal. Other options are to train select field staff or management staff who can be coaches, or to use computer-based training modules (CBT). CBT modules can be set up on the Internet as a web-based application, as done in many education settings. Clinicians can access the training modules as a way to review their learning or as a remedial exercise. If CBT is not available from the vendor, the development of CBT can be costly and may not be an option for all agencies.

EVALUATION

"An evaluation of a health informatics system is needed not only to prove its value, but also to determine if the system is doing what was originally intended" (Lorenzi et al., 1995, p. 388). In the aftermath of the implementation, the team is likely to hear mixed messages as to the success of the project. The organization needs to have objective data on the outcomes of the project. The lack of baseline data can jeopardize the evaluation (Lorenzi et al., 1995). This suggests that the evaluation has to be built in from the beginning. The stated goals and objectives for the automated system are starting points.

The requirements document or the cost-benefit analysis both provide relevant areas for evaluation. The achievement of any projected efficiency in business operations, such as reduced clerical staff, elimination of printing, is quantifiable. Improvement in regulatory compliance is measurable as well. Examples are expedited billing and return of signed physician orders, timely performance of recertifications, and timely submission of OASIS data.

A second area for consideration is system performance. This area significantly impacts the organization and the users. Possible measures of system performance are data processing time on the mobile computers (also a factor in staff satisfaction); length of time of modem transmissions; communication failures; timely data transmission from the field to the client-server or mainframe; database corruption; help-desk response time; and problem resolution. The team should receive routine reports on the number of reported problems and documented resolutions called-in to the help-desk and/or vendor.

The acceptance of computer technology by the clinical staff is a major concern in implementing an automated system. The perceived ease of use, usefulness (Dillon, McDowell, Salimian, & Conklin, 1998), and perceived efficiencies are measures of user satisfaction. This data can be gathered through various means such as a user survey, clinical staff turnover rates, and as part of the exit interview process. The success of the training is another useful measure and can be reported based on training evaluations and the scores from homework exercises.

SUMMARY

The use of computers by clinicians in home health care is relatively recent. Information technology has not been used to its maximum potential, but with the onset of PPS, the environment is poised for change. The management of clinical data and business processes require sophisticated systems that can analyze an agency's case-mix, utilization, and clinical outcomes in relation to reimbursement rates.

Nurses are at the heart of home care. Their ability to use systems in their clinical practice may well be the only means to survive in a capitated environment. It matters how systems are introduced into the home care setting, the data that is captured in the field, and how that data is managed. Nurses who take on the responsibility to work with information technology have a strategic role in the ultimate outcome.

REFERENCES

Dillon, T., McDowell, D., Salimian, F., & Conklin, D. (1998). Perceived ease of use and usefulness of bedside-computer systems. *Computers in Nursing, 16*(3), 151–156.

Dombi, W., & St. Pierre, M. (1999). Interim payment system and risk management. *Caring, 18*(6), 34–8.

Geraci, E. (1997). Computers in home care: Application of change theory. *Computers in Nursing, 15*(4), 199–205.

Lorenzi, N. M., Riley, R. T., Ball, M. J., & Douglas, J. V. (1995). *Transforming health care through information: Case studies.* New York: Springer-Verlag.

Mallard, C., & Mitchell, R. (1998). Two approaches to developing a computer-based patient record for home health care. *Home Health Care Manage Practice, 10*(6), 29–37.

Martin, K., & Scheet, N. J. (1992). *The OMAHA System: Applications for community health nursing.* Philadelphia: W. B. Saunders Company.

McSpedon, C. (1999). The transition to prospective payment changes the face of home care. *Managed Care Interface, 12*(5), 77–80, 82–3.

Mead, C. (1995). Pen-based computing and homecare: Perfect fit or hype? *Buyers Guide.* Spring.

Mikos, C., & Koch, L. (1999). The legal considerations surrounding OASIS (Outcome Assessment and Information Set) reporting requirements. *Caring, 18*(3), 20–3.

Saba, V. K. (1997). Why the home health care classification is a recognized nursing nomenclature. *Computers in Nursing, 15*(2S), S69–S76.

St. Pierre, M. (1999). A look to the future: Home health. *Caring, 18*(3), 16–19.

Shaughnessy, P., Crisler, K., Schlenker, R., Arnold, A., Kramer, A., Powell, M., & Hittle, D. (1994). Measuring and assuring the quality of home health care. *Health Care Financing Review, 16*(1), 35–67.

Whitten, J. L., & Bentley, L. D. (1998). *Systems analysis and design methods.* Boston: Irwin McGraw-Hill.

14

Informatics and Education:
The Start of a Discussion
James P. Turley

The purpose of this chapter is not to provide an answer to what the role of education should be for informatics as a whole (Hasman, Albert, Wainwright, Klar, & Sosa, 1995) and nursing informatics in particular. Rather the purpose of this chapter is to start that discussion. Worldwide there are a number of educational programs that focus on informatics. Lest we forget, not all of these programs are health related. There are programs that focus on "informatics" as an independent science that involves the modeling of knowledge. The University of Michigan, School of Information Science offers such a program in the United States Similar programs exist in Europe and Australia.

Indeed whether we focus on Health Informatics, Nursing Informatics, Medical Informatics, or some other "hyphenated" informatics, we must be clear about the definition of informatics which is being addressed. Every educational program is explicitly or implicitly based on an informatics definition. The importance of that definition in defining the premises, scope, organization, and the outcomes of the educational program cannot be underestimated. While we cannot spend time in this chapter to focus on the definitions of informatics, health informatics, or nursing informatics, we will attempt to be cognizant of the impact of those definitions on the educational programs and models presented in this chapter.

The chapter will examine the types and levels of educational programs that are currently available, the relation of those programs to the health professions, with a special focus on nursing, and some suggestions as to what the future might be for informatics education and the impact on informated practice[1]. We know that both the conceptual development of informatics and the technology that it interacts with are in rapid transition. The result is that we should expect rapid changes and transitions in the educational programs related to informatics as well. Hence, everything said may be out of date by the time it gets to print.

CURRENT PROGRAMS

In the health-related area of informatics, the vast majority of programs exist within discipline schools. In the United States, we find the greatest number of programs in Schools of Medicine. The second largest number of programs is in Schools of Nursing. The remainder of the programs tend to be less concentrated, such as programs in Schools of Dentistry, Allied Health Science, and other schools. This concentration of schools is less true outside of the United States where educational programs are more widely distributed throughout the university and where educational programs tend to be less insular in organizational structure.

When informatics programs sit within discipline schools they have a tendency to reflect the domain knowledge of that discipline and to be structured to meet the specific needs of that discipline. Many of the programs located within discipline schools require that students have the discipline credential as part of the admission process. This is particularly true of nursing programs that require a degree in nursing as part of the admission process. Medical informatics programs are more varied. Some of the programs have a focus on medicine or even a sub-discipline of medicine as the programs may be housed in Departments of Internal Medicine, Pathology, Radiology, etc. Other programs, housed in medical schools, have deliberately made an outreach to other health disciplines. The University of Minnesota has a long history of inviting nurses, health educators, veterinarians, and others to join physicians in their program in Health Computer Sciences located in the Medical School. More recently, the University of Missouri-Columbia, School of Medicine, Department of Health

---

[1] The process of understanding that the core of any professional practice is determined by the data, information, knowledge, and thought processes used in the planning, delivery, and evaluation of care. Skills are the processes used to gain, synthesize, and apply the data, information, and knowledge.

Management and Informatics has recruited students from a wide range of health disciplines. Other programs allow a different range of opportunities based on the unique qualifications of each student applying to the program.

By virtue of being included in a discipline school, many informatics programs have a focus on the discipline knowledge of that school. Hence, programs in schools of nursing share a focus on nursing knowledge as a central aspect of the program. For programs in schools of medicine, the issue can become more complex as to whether the program will focus on the science of medicine as a whole or will focus on the sub-discipline that gave the initial rise to the program. While not always the case, it is possible for programs associated with radiology departments to have a special focus on the issues of image compression and the transmission of large-scale files associated with radiographic images. Programs associated with internal medicine are more likely to focus on the decision-making needs of the clinician. Here the physician is likely to have access to large amounts of data that could be associated with a multitude of possible diseases. There is a felt need to improve decision making and make it more efficient. This decision making may be associated with disease diagnosis, drug therapies, or diagnostic test ordering. These are general-purpose problems that can be generalized to other areas of care and to other professions. Thus, these departments seem to have a special place in the history and research into informatics problems.

LEVELS OF EDUCATION

When we discuss education in informatics, it is often assumed that we are referring to graduate education. Indeed when we think about education and nursing informatics the University of Utah, the University of Maryland and New York University, all of which have graduate programs in nursing informatics come to mind. However, nursing has a long history of considering the inclusion of informatics education at the undergraduate level. Travis and Brennan (1998) and Grobe (1988) among others have written on the need for the inclusion of informatics concepts into the basic programs of nursing. Similar discussions can be found in medicine (Espino, & Levine,

1998; McGowan, Raszka, Light, Magrane, O'Malley, & Bertsch, 1998). There is increasing recognition that informatics information must be included into the basic programs of all the health professions. The International Medical Informatics Association (IMIA) has recognized this need quite explicitly in their draft recommendations (IMIA, 1999). The IMIA recommendations focus on the need for future clinicians to be knowledgeable users of information and information technology throughout their education and leading on into their practice. The role of educational institutions to create "informated practitioners" is early in its history.

The Association of American Medical Colleges (AAMC) (AAMC, 1998) operation with the American Medical Informatics Association (AMIA) has drafted guidelines that are expected to be included in the curriculum of all medical colleges in the future. These guidelines have a strong focus on technical skills in the area of knowledge use and acquisition, which can be argued to the most transient form of informatics knowledge. However, this is at least the beginning recognition of the need for the inclusion of informatics at all levels of education from the basic professional education to the extended needs of the life-long learner. The AAMC document does recognize that the needs of learners change at different points in their careers as the demands of the roles which clinicians adopt change.

The result is a need to examine at least three levels of education:

1. that occurring in a basic program,
2. education occurring in a post-basic or graduate program, and
3. life-long learning or continuing education.

Post-basic education has two categories:

1. informatics-focused education, and
2. post-basic education where informatics is an ancillary component of the educational program.

Continuing education also breaks into two discrete forms:

1. one that is initiated by the individual, and
2. education initiated by the employing institution.

BASIC PROGRAM INFORMATICS EDUCATION

Like the AAMC guidelines, much of the literature related to the inclusion of informatics into the basic educational programs tends to focus on the instrumental aspects of informatics education. Traditionally, these instrumental aspects have focused on issues of "computer literacy" or technology in the basic programs. Carty and Rosenfeld (1997) assessed the status of technology in the U.S. nursing education programs. At the same time, Nelson and Anton (1997) assessed the organizational need for technology utilization in clinical or academic health care organizations. There is a long history of this type of technology assessment in nursing education as well as the other health professions (Cammann, Michel, Uhlmann, & Orlow, 1992; Davis, Hassett, 1994; Rizzolo, 1994). Before the assessment of computer literacy, there was a long period of assessing nursing attitudes toward computers and computing. This chapter will argue that there are four major categories of information which should be contained in informatics programs:

1. understanding the data,
2. combining data, information, and knowledge,
3. decision making, and
4. technology.

This is important because in nursing and medicine as well, there has been a period of confusing technology with informatics. Nursing informatics definitions such as those by Graves and Corcoran (1989) and Turley (1996) have not generally included computer literacy as part of the definition. Rather the definitions have assumed that the technology was part of the background or the field in which the definition was developed. Most of the important work in nursing informatics is not completely dependent on computer technology. However, the work of informatics is made much easier and more efficient by the use of computer technology. Work in taxonomy development could be done without the use of computers. However, the work would be tedious and painfully slow. Other aspects of informatics work such as the organization and display of clinical data are indeed fully dependent on computer technology. Think of graphical data display—can you imagine a PET scan or a MRI without access to a computer? But even in these cases where the computer is integral to this type of informatics work, issues of computer literacy do not come to the foreground. Issues of computer literacy are part of the technological assumptions of working in the late 20th century. These issues of computer literacy occur, as they occur with all working people. Manufacturing uses computerized machinery; supermarkets have computer-based scanning systems, automobiles contain entire computer networks. There are function issues, yes. But these are simply job-task requirements to function in a technical environment.

If informatics is not the same as computer literacy, what is indeed the role of informatics in the basic education program? A number of suggestions have been made by AAMC (1998), Travis and Brennan (1998), Grobe (1988), IMIA (1999), and others. In its summary of issues, IMIA (1999, p. 11) suggests that the goal is "to focus on the processing of data, information and knowledge in healthcare and medicine with a strong focus on the need for profound knowledge and skills of health and medical informatics, of mathematics, as well as of theoretical, practical and technical informatics/computer science." Likewise, AAMC (1998) states that the educational premise is "To support healthcare, life-long learning, education, research and management, medical students should be able, at the time of graduation, to utilize biomedical information for: formulating problems; arriving at strategies for solutions; collecting, critiquing and analyzing information; taking action based on findings; and communicating and documenting these processes and the results."

Both the IMIA and AAMC papers focus on the need to assist students in the accessing of relevant data, aggregate that data into information, combine that information with knowledge, and assist in the decision-making process. This is very different than computer literacy, thought it does assume computer literacy. Working in today's health care environment, the issue is not usually a lack of data but rather an excess of data. Many of the instruments used in contemporary health care supply a never-ending supply of data. Telemetry systems supply vital signs and physiologic monitoring data in a way that overwhelms the ability of the clinician to use the data. In neonatal intensive care units (NICUs), clinicians are not only saturated by the continuous readout of data, but they are also oversaturated by the continuous demand of alarms for attention. One of the sure ways to tell that a clinician is a novice in this area is that he/she rapidly responds to all alarms. One of the first informatics issues is then to understand the relative importance of data points. The ability to "filter out" data and learn which data points to pay attention to is a complex task and one that is not formally taught. By participating in the culture of a clinical site, clinicians of all types teach the students of their own profession as well as students of other professions the culturally acceptable response to certain types of data and information.

The process of learning to interpret data streams probably should be seen as one of the critical informatics tasks that clinicians learn early on in their careers. The *meaning* of the data stream is often taught as part of the didactic program. The *response to* or the *usefulness* of the data streams is often taught in the clinical portions of the educational process.

Likewise, the formal aspects of data access are often taught as part of the basic educational program. This is true whether the data source is the patient, a lab report, information gathered from a parent, or how to access the literature to gain information. The importance of data gathering becomes more apparent when the task is to combine data from several sources for the purpose of making a diagnostic statement or hypothesis. Data cannot stand on its own importance. Data is important as it is compared with data from other sources, or other times. Knowing how to combine data into information and knowing what data at what time *should be* combined is often the second major informatics task. While this task is often achieved in a basic clinical program, clinical programs usually do not help their students by giving them an introduction to the types and styles of information processing. Knowledge of the different decision-making theories (Elstein, & Shulman, 1978), with their assumptions, strengths, and weaknesses could easily improve the efficiency of the decision-making process for beginning clinicians.

Once the decision-making process is understood by the basic student, then the student can be exposed to decision support systems. Like decision making itself, decision support systems are based on different models (Tan, 1998). Decision support can be used to assist the student to learn the process that is being assisted. Smith, Obradovich, Heintz, Guerkin, Rudmann, et al. (1998) have described the process of using decision support as a tutorial process, rather than using it to replace the decision making of the clinician. When the decision support system replaces the clinician's decision making, the clinician loses the ability to make the decision independently and is at a loss when the decision support is not available. Whereas if the clinician's decision making has been monitored and supported, the clinician learns more about the domain and the decision-making process and is easily able to function when the support system is not available.

Closely linked to data and clinical decision making are issues of taxonomy and taxonomic structure. Each of the health professions has invested a great amount of time in developing or adapting standardized languages. This is not to imply that the average clinician *speaks* any of the standardized languages. However, we know that if a physician wants to be paid, information about a client visit must be able to be formalized into ICD-9, ICD-9-CM, or ICD-10 codes along with CPT-4 codes. Nursing has a growing number of standardized codes which started with NANDA and have continued to progress. Werley (Werley & Lang, 1988) has argued for years about the need to adopt a Nursing Minimum Data Set (NMDS) in the United States. The NMDS is based on a set of standardized codes. Other countries such as Australia and Belgium are using standardized taxonomies to collect nurse-sensitive data on many if not all of their patients. The importance of taxonomy development in health care cannot be underestimated. Taxonomy development is the basis by which clinicians from different agencies, different areas, and even different countries, speaking different languages form a mechanism for clear and unambiguous communication not only within their discipline but also to communicate with other disciplines. Yet the discussion of taxonomies and standardized languages tends to be one of the components universally missing from the basic programs in health care.

Communication is often presented in basic programs as communication between the patient/client and the clinician, and assumes a physical presence. There needs to be a greater discussion of the importance of communication within and among disciplines (Turley, 2000) and how disciplines relate to communication with clients. The impact of technology in health care: e-mail, telehealth, and remote presence increase the complexity of communication. Such a consideration is beyond the scope of the present discussion.

Lastly, basic students should be knowledgeable about the technology that is being used in health care. This is not the same as functional literacy. Rather, the student should know enough about the technology to know the strengths, weaknesses, and limits of the technology. Currently, we often see that students make impossible requests of technology or fail to use the technology to the limits that it is capable, even though they have a basic literacy with the technology. While they have functional literacy, they do not understand how the technology functions, and hence do not know what they can expect of that technology. Nowhere is that more clearly seen than in student utilization of the Internet. Without understanding the structure and functioning of the Internet, search-engines and associated technology, students frequently *"get lost" in cyberspace* and cannot return to the Web-site a day later. Researchers are alarmed to find out that the Web-site they cited in an article last week is no longer available as a reference. Stability of structure and information is not a hallmark of the Internet and therefore it should be no surprise to find the Internet volatile. Knowledge of the technology does not guarantee literacy anymore than perceived literacy implies an understanding of the technology.

What is the role of informatics education in a basic education program? This discussion would suggest that the student should understand data, information, and knowledge. The student should understand how to combine data, information, and knowledge. This understanding comes to a focal point in the process of decision making. The student should understand different theoretical processes for decision making and the implication of the different models for the development of decision support systems. With this knowledge, the student will be able to understand how to use decision support systems and to understand the impact of decision support systems on how the student builds a model of clinical knowledge for the student's own clinical application. Issues of communication and technology are becoming increasingly intertwined. As these become part of the everyday clinical settings, students must become increasingly knowledgeable about communication, its process, its outcomes, and metrics for the understanding of each component of communication. Technology will be an ever-changing floor that will increasingly be used to support the entire health care process. Students who do not understand that technology will not be able to use it appropriately or effectively.

POST-BASIC PROGRAM INFORMATICS EDUCATION

Post-basic education takes many forms in different countries. The issues for post-basic program education are similar whether we are discussing a master's degree, a certificate, a graduate diploma, a post-doc, or some other formal educational program. For our purposes, post-basic education will be divided into two categories:

1. informatics focused education, and
2. post-basic education where informatics is ancillary or support to the basic reason for the education.

Post-basic Informatics Focused Education

The majority of informatics-focused programs exist within discipline schools. The impact of being within a discipline school has been discussed above. Indeed, as we see the importance of communication in health care and the impact of informatics in the future development of communication, one of the major questions is whether a discipline centric view of informatics is really useful. This is a question that we will address later. First, given our assumptions about what informatics content has been included in the basic program, the emphasis turns on what should be the focus of informatics in the post-basic program when informatics itself is the focus of the program.

Health care has contained a historically fractured past. There are a number of disciplines. Each health care discipline has in turn created its own set of sub-disciplines. The sub-disciplines have been created on the basis of domain knowledges, skill sets, and politics. The result has been that the delivery of health care is as fractured as the sub-disciplines that have been created to deliver it. The early stage of health informatics has mirrored the fractional division of the sub-disciplines. Hence we have had informatics programs started in departments of radiology and internal medicine that have not sought any common core. We have had dental informatics programs that have had no alliance with programs in medicine and nursing. In a worst-case scenario, we have seen separate programs in health informatics started in separate schools on the same campus with little or no communication between them.

If communication is a critical element to be supported by informatics, then communication must be seen as a critical element of informatics itself. The development of communication as a central element in informatics is being seen in definitions of informatics (Turley, 2000; IMIA, 1999). In order for informatics to function, it must overcome the divisions that have traditionally separated health care disciplines and sub-disciplines. The advent of "patient centered" care implies that the functions of those in service to health must be subordinated to the needs of the patient or client. As we move into the notion of patient centered practice, we must also move into the model of informated practice.

The person focusing on informatics must focus on developing, applying, and testing informatics components to insure that those with a basic informatics education have data, information, and knowledge systems that indeed function in the way they are indented by the clinician users. This implies that the systems and/or structures must be useful within disciplines and across disciplines. In our complex health care environment, it is increasingly the issue that we must be aware of the cross-discipline aspects. The following figure gives some structure to the discussion.

Knowledge Generator		Nursing	Medicine	Social Work	Dentistry	Insurance	Health Planner
User or Purpose for the Data	Nursing Communication	X					
	Medical Communication		X				
	Social Workers Com.			X			
	Dental Communication				X		
	Case Managers Com.						
	Quality Managers Com.		.				
	Patient/Client Com.						

FIGURE 14.1 Data Source vs. User or Purpose of Data. Information & Knowledge.

When informatics education programs reside within a discipline school, the focus on the program seems to run on the diagonal as marked by the "X." Thus nursing programs worry about communication within nursing, medicine within medicine, etc. If we examine the four components that we noted in the basic informatics education:

1. understanding the data,
2. combining data, information, and knowledge,
3. decision making, and
4. technology, we find a grid that is familiar to many of the discipline informatics programs.

Each program will vary to some degree as to how they will implement the grid and the amount of importance that will be given to each cell or sub-cell in the grid. Examples will be given for nursing but could apply to any health discipline. The example is not meant to be exhaustive but rather indicative.

Some aspects become clear when looking at such a list. The first is that not every aspect of informatics will be able to be covered in every program. The range and complexity of the material indicates that there will need to be a degree of concentration and focus. Indeed when we look at the curriculum of different nursing informatics programs, we see that this is clearly happening.

What also becomes clear from Figure 14.1 is that not all information is communicated within a discipline. Indeed, it may be that the majority of health information is communicated across discipline boundaries. Traditionally this has been an area of weakness in most informatics programs. When nursing programs focus only on the nursing domain, the concern has been for the communication of phenomena of concern to nursing to other nurses. Yet the reality of contemporary health care is that it "takes a team" to deliver care. When disciplines focus on the communication of issues within the discipline, that may be good, but it is not serving the needs of the patient for the other members that make up the health care team. One need only look at the use of nursing taxonomies when they are addressed to other members of the health care team. Does that mean that the phenomena described in these taxonomies are of no use? Hardly. The work of Henry, Warren, Lange, and Button (1998) have

TABLE 14.1 Category and Possible Content for an Informatics Educational Program

Category	Possible content
Data	
Taxonomy & Nomenclature[1]	• NANDA • Nursing Interventions Classification System/Nursing Outcomes Classification System • Nursing Management Minimum Data Set • Home Health Care Classifications • Omaha System • Patient Care Data Set • Perioperative Nursing Dataset • SNOMED / RT
Combining data information and knowledge	
Development of Minimum Data Sets	• US-NMDS • Community Nursing Minimum Data Set • Nursing Management Data Set
Knowledge Induction	• Mental Models of data, information • ARKS • Data Mining
Decision making in nursing	
Decision models	• Information Processing • LENS • Judgment
Decision Support Systems	• Technology of Decision Support • Examples of Decision Support • Florence Nightingale

TABLE 14.1 *(continued)*

Category	Possible content
Federal guidelines	• HIPAA • HCFA • AHCPR
Technology	
Database	• Relational • Network • Hierarchical • Object oriented
Communication	• H 323 Internet Video • H 320 Interactive TV • T 120 White Board
Standards Organizations	• CPRI • DICOM • CEN-TC-251 • ASTM
Ubiquitous computing	• Human Computer Interface • Imbedded Systems • Augmented Reality

¹ ANA Nursing Classification Systems

documented that these nurse-sensitive phenomenon are not well-documented in the other taxonomies. Rather, it is clear that these taxonomies have been developed in isolation from other health care team members and the meaning and structure of the phenomena have not been communicated to the other team members. As a result, the developed taxonomies do not achieve their goal of communicated new and vital phenomena in a way that can be understood by the other health care team members.

The goal of post-basic informatics programs is to develop systems that work. These systems must occur at all four of the identified levels. Taxonomies and nomenclatures must achieve their communication goals. To achieve this, they cannot be developed in isolation from all of the people and groups who will use them. This is the beginning of a recognition for a trans-disciplinary approach to informatics education in post-basic education. As an aside, this is not a demand that all health care workers should *speak NANDA*; rather it is recognition that no one should *speak NANDA*. NANDA or one of the other taxonomies should act as a structured, standardized language for the communication of information. Information recorded in the Electronic Health Record (EHR) should be mapped to a standardized language to allow unambiguous communication. Physicians and nurse-practitioners do not speak ICD-9-CM or CPT-4, yet information in their records are mapped to these standardized languages in order to allow for correct billing. The use of taxonomies and structured languages is that they can be used for unambiguous communication. The EHR allows the mapping to occur in a much more convenient way than when "coders" had to do the job manually.

When the basic data level is not clear, then as we move up through data combination and decision support, there is a continued lack of clarity. For those who are involved in post-basic informatics programs, their goal must be to design in the communication and the clarity. They must understand how the data, information, and knowledge is designed and structured for the disciplines that are working together in the health care enterprise. Obviously, this is more easily done when they study together, than if each group is in a solo based program.

The role of the consumer of health care is changing. With the advent of the Internet and Web-based materials, the consumers of health care have access to increasing amounts of health care knowledge of variable quality. The impact of this change on health informatics education is not well understood. If Tom Ferguson (1999) is to be believed, the impact will increase rapidly.

So again, what is the role of post-basic informatics education? The answer is that people who have post-basic informatics education should be in the process of identifying, developing, and implementing the components which will improve the communication among health care personnel. These may take different forms depending on the level that the person is working in. These aspects can take place within the area of a single domain knowledge before being integrated into functions with other health care providers.

Table 14.2 is not meant to be an exhaustive list of components for an educational program, rather it is an example of how the outline could be used to drive a program from a discipline specific model to one which will meet the needs and demands of a trans-disciplinary program which reflects the needs of health care as it is delivered.

Post-basic Non-Informatics Focused Education

Post-basic non-informatics focused education takes a wide variety of presentations. Examples could include: residency training programs, internships, externships, graduate degree programs, certificates, graduate diplomas, and other programs. Different disciplines and different countries make use of each of these types of programs in ways that meet the health care needs of the population being served. In discussing the needs for an Internal Medicine Informatics curriculum, Weiner and Osheroff (1997) discussed the need for topics that focus on computer literacy and only minimal knowledge that would be directly related to informatics. Another is the ambitious Nightingale program in Europe to bring nursing informatics education to over 3,000 nurses (Nightingale, 1999). Protti and Anglin (1992) have argued for a variety of health informatics programs and indeed for a taxonomy that would describe each type of program. In addition, the AAMC (1998) report recognized the need for lifelong learners, those who were included in ongoing education and those who were seeking continuing education.

When people are enrolled in post-basic non-informatics focused education, the issue that is most clear is that informatics education is not the primary focus of the program. The goals of that program, be it a clinical program such as a nurse-practitioner program or an oncology residency or an academic program such as epidemiology, are the primary goals of the student. Informatics should provide a supporting role. At this time, we will assume that the student has had exposure to informatics in his/her basic program. If not, remedial work will be required.

The supporting role for informatics will be directed by the goals of the program in conjunction with the goals of the student. Increasingly, those goals are focusing on the computational needs in the delivery of health care. From the supporting role, the focus should be on how people are users of the informatics. Some people

TABLE 14.2 Category and Possible Content for an Informatics Educational Program in a Trans-disciplinary Environment

Category	Intra-discipline	Trans-discipline
Data		
Taxonomy & Nomenclature[1]	• Develop appropriate taxonomies	• Link to other taxonomies
Combining data information and knowledge		
Development of Minimum Data Sets	• US-NMDS • Community Nursing Minimum Data Set • Nursing Management Data Set	• Coordinate with other data sets, e.g., UB-92, Hospital Discharge Data Set, etc.
Knowledge Induction	• Mental Models • ARKS • Data Mining	• Compare disciplines • information models • Coordinate use of data into Data Warehouse • Use aggregate clinical knowledge to create care paths
Decision Making		
Decision models	• Information processing • LENS • Judgment	• Apply decision model to unique and cooperative decisions
Decision Support Systems	• Technology of Decision Support • Examples of Decision Support • Florence Nightingale	• Integrate decision support systems to address all client needs • Coordinate decisions for comprehensive care

TABLE 14.2 *(continued)*

Category	Intra-discipline	Trans-discipline
Federal guidelines		• HIPAA • HCFA • AHCPR
Technology		
Database	• Relational • Network • Hierarchical • Object oriented	• Decide on appropriate technology to achieve project goal
Communication	• H 323 Internet Video • H 320 Interactive TV • T 120 White Board	• Determine the impact of communication technology on clinical practice
Standards Organizations	• CPRI • DICOM • CEN-TC-251 • ASTM	• Be certain that choices address industry standards
Ubiquitous computing	• Interface Design • Imbedded Systems • Augmented Reality	• Compare discipline display needs • Monitor industry and technology trends[2] • Creating computationally efficient data

[2] e.g. Elliott, J. (1999). Nine Hot Technology Trends

will be users of information systems, some will be users of taxonomies, some will apply mental models of data to specific domains, some will look at the use of information systems under controlled circumstances, and others will be involved with the implementation of informatics systems and structures within their environments. The important issue is for health informatics programs to maintain the structural flexibility to meet the needs of these students.

Another issue related to the post-basic informatics educational needs of students is that the students themselves have a wide variety of backgrounds. For the educational programs to be efficient as well as effective, the programs must allow the students to place into the program based on the student's demonstrated expertise rather than assuming a "one size fits all" approach to the educational program. Education in the health arena does not have a history of excessive flexibility. Many educational programs have been highly structured with long lists of stated prerequisites that allow students to move through the program in only one way. Students have learned much about informatics on their own; they will need to build on their existing knowledge to most efficiently gain the knowledge and skills they need in their post-basic education.

If programs are based on the assumptions of adult learning and recognize that the students seeking post-basic education are highly motivated, programs can maintain high quality and still have flexibility. This will require customization of the programs to the needs of the individual student and also be based on the expertise that the student brings to the program. The process requires more student advising and assessment than is traditionally done, but the results can be highly customized to the needs of the student at the time. The need for customization is widely recognized in our society and must become a major component of higher education (Friedman, 1999).

The role of informatics in post-basic education where informatics is not the main focus of the program must be mercurial. As informatics becomes an increasing focus in the delivery of health care, the needs of the students will be more varied and more applied. Programs will need to adapt to the changing needs of the students and the changing needs of the health care environment. Yet, flexibility is not historically a trademark of health care education.

CONTINUING EDUCATION

The role of continuing education in health care has had a varied history. In some states and for some professions, this is a requirement of continued certification. In other areas, there is no formal requirement for continued education, but recognition that it is simply part of the professional role to stay current on new developments in the field.

Others seek out continuing education for an increase in domain knowledge. For these people, the informatics domain knowledge can be either applied or more pure. Some professional's use continuing education as a means of "testing the waters" before moving into a post-basic education program. Historically, there has been a separation between education provided in academic programs and that provided in continuing education. As programs move toward Web-based education, it is more efficient to take materials developed for a course program and reposition those materials in smaller modules for continuing education. When students move into a program that recognize their previous knowledge bases, then continuing education feeds directly into the post-basic education making the claim of "lifelong learning" a true reality.

The role of continuing education is part of a larger set of professional questions and standards. As an emerging discipline in a rapidly changing health care market, it would seem that informatics has a special responsibility in this area. However, this is a topic that demands further discussion at another time.

SUMMARY

As stated in the beginning, the goal of this chapter was not to answer questions but rather to begin a discussion on the role of education and informatics. Informatics is changing rapidly. The technology with which it is associated is changing even more rapidly. Health care is moving with its own rate of change. As the three areas intersect, it is difficult to view with any clarity what the result will be in the near or distant future. We know that some will hold onto the past and declare that any change will hamper the quality of health care that was clearly better in the past. Others will look forward and say that we are evolving into a totally new model of health care that will create new possibilities and opportunities. We can be certain that things will not stay the same.

The role and function of informatics is tied to communication. Communication is a volatile area. Clear and unambiguous communication does not mean that we will like the content of what is being communicated. However, without clear communication we will never understand the content of what is being communicated.

The role of the health care providers and the role of the client will change dramatically in an area where "high bandwidth communication" is ubiquitous. Will the consumer really appreciate being involved in all aspects of their health care? Will care providers be able to practice when the consumers have better access to information than the providers have? Can we develop new paradigms for cooperative health care? All of these are possible results of the rise in informatics. How we choose to educate our professions, our practitioners, our society, and ourselves remains to be seen. It will be an interesting process. Let's continue the discussion.

REFERENCES

AAMC (1998). Medical school objectives project: Medical informatics objectives. URL: *http://www.aamc.org/meded/msop/informat.htm* (accessed 9/18/99).

ANA. Nursing Classification Systems. URL: *http://www.ana.org/nidsec/classlst.htm* (accessed 9/20/99)

Cammann, H., Michel, J., Uhlmann, G., & Orlow, W. (1992). Computer programs in support of teaching medical informatics with particular reference to medical signal processing. In Lun, K.C., Degoulet, P., Piemme, T.E., Rienhoff, O. (Eds.), *MEDINFO 92: Proceedings of the Seventh World Congress on medical Informatics.* New York: North-Holland.

Carty, B., & Rosenfeld, P. (1997). The information age: The status of technology in nursing education programs in the United States. In Gerden, U., Tallberg, M., Wainwright, P. (Eds.), Nursing Informatics: *The Impact of Nursing Knowledge on Health Care Informatics.* Washington, DC: IOS Press.

Davis, K. E., & Hassett, M. M. (1994). Meting communication needs with an electronic bulletin board. In Grobe, S. J., Pluyter-Wenting, E. S. P. (Eds.), *Nursing Informatics: An International Overview for Nursing in a Technological Era.* New York: Elsevier.

Elliott, J. (1999). Nine hot technology trends. *Healthcare Informatics Online.* (Feb. 1999). URL: *http://www.healthcare-informatics.com/issues/1999/02_99/nine.htm* (accessed 9/20/99).

Elstein, A. S., & Shulman, L. S. (1978). *Medical problem solving: An analysis of clinical reasoning.* Boston: Harvard University Press.

Espino, J., & Levine, M. G. (1998). An overview of the medical informatics curriculum in medical schools. *A Paradigm Shift in Health Care Information Systems.* Bethesda, MD: AMIA.

Ferguson, T. (1999). Ferguson Report. URL: *http://ferguson-report.*

sparklist.com (accessed 9/21/99).

Friedman, T. L. (1999). *The lexus and the olive tree: Understanding globalization.* New York: Farrar Straus & Giroux.

Graves, J. R., & Corcoran, S. A. (1989). The study of nursing informatics. *Image: Journal of Nursing Scholarship,* 1989, 21, 227–31.

Grobe, S. J. (1988). Nursing informatics competencies for nurse educators and researchers. In: *Preparing nurses for using information systems: recommended informatics competencies.* National League for Nursing Publications. NLN PUBL ** 1988 #14–2234 (pp. 25–40).

Hasman, A., Albert, A., Wainwright, P., Klar, R., & Sosa, M. (1995). *Education and training in health informatics in Europe.* Washington, DC: IOS Press.

Henry, S. B., Warren, J. J., Lange, L., & Button, P. (1998). A review of major nursing vocabularies and the extent to which they have the characteristics required for implementation in computer-based systems. *J Am Med Inform Assoc,* Jul–Aug, 5, (4), 321–8. Review.

IMIA (1999). Recommendations of the International Medical Informatics Association (IMIA) on Education in Health and Medical Informatics. URL: *http://www.med.uni-heidelberg.de/mi* (accessed 9/18/99).

McGowan, J. J., Raszka, W., Light, J., Magrane, D., O'Malley, D., & Bertsch, T. (1998). A vertical curriculum to teach the knowledge, skill and attitudes of medical informatics. *A Paradigm Shift in Health Care Information Systems.* Bethesda, MD: AMIA.

Nelson, R., & Anton, R. (1997). Organizational diagnosis of computer and information learning needs: The process and the product. In Gerden, U., Tallberg, M., Wainwright, P. (Eds.), Nursing Informatics: *The Impact of Nursing Knowledge on Health Care Informatics.* Washington, DC: IOS Press.

Nightingale Project. (1999). URL: *http://www.sgim.org/meetings/am20/ws/infocurric. html* (accessed 9/20/99).

Protti, D. J., & Anglin, C. R. (1992). The continuum of health informatics education: where do the existing curricula fit? In Lun, K. C., Degoulet, P., Piemme, T. E., Rienhoff, O. (Eds.), *MEDINFO 92: Proceedings of the Seventh World Congress on medical Informatics.* New York: North-Holland.

Rizzolo, M. A. (1994). Multimedia patient case study simulations: Considerations for their evaluation and use. In Grobe, S. J., Pluyter-Wenting, E. S. P. (Eds.), *Nursing Informatics: An International*

Overview for Nursing in a Technological Era. New York: Elsevier.
Smith, P. J., Obradovich, J., Heintz, Guerlain, S., Rudmann, S., Strohm, P., Smith, J. W., Svirbely, J., & Sachs, L. (1998). Successful use of an expert system to teach diagnostic reasoning for antibody identification. *Proceedings of the Fourth International Conference on Intelligent Tutoring Systems. San Antonio, Texas, August 16–19, 354–363.* URL: *http://www-iwse.eng.ohio-state.edu/~PJSmith/ITS98.htm* (accessed 9/22/99).
Tan, J. K. (1998). *Health decision support systems.* Gaithersburg, MD: Aspen.
Travis, L., & Brennan, P. F. (1998). Information science for the future: an innovative nursing informatics curriculum. *Journal of Nursing Education, 37*(4), 162–8.
Turley, J. P. (1996). Toward a model of nursing informatics. *Image: Journal of Nursing Scholarship, 1997; 28*(4), 229–32.
Turley, J. P. (2000). Toward an integrated view of health informatics. *Nursing Informatics 2000* (in press).
Weiner, M., & Osheroff, G. (1997). Designing an informatics curriculum in residency training. URL: *http://www.sgim.org/meetings/am20/ws/infocurric.html* (accessed 9/21/99).
Werley, H., & Lang, N. (1988). *Identification of the nursing minimum data set.* New York : Springer.

Appendix
Web URL Locations

URL	Organizations	Chapter
http://nursingworld.org/nidsec/index.htm	American Nurses Association NIDSEC	Chapter 1
http://www.cpri.org	Computer-based Patient Record Institute	Chapter 1
http://ferguson-report.sparklist.com	Ferguson Report.	Chapter 1
http://www.dol.gov	Department of Labor	Chapter 1
http:/www.nita.doc.gov	Dept. of Commerce, "Falling through the Net"	Chapter 1
http://www.imia.org/wg1	International Medical Informatics Association	Chapter 2
http://www.ana.org/ancc/certify/catalogs/1998 /inform98/infomat.htm.	American Nurses Credentialing Center—ANCC Informatics Nurse Certification Catalog	Chapter 2
http://www.ana.org/acnn/exams.htm	American Nurses Credentialing Center— Certification Exam Results	Chapter 2
http://www.nursingworld.org/tan/99janfeb/ kaleid.htm.	American Nurses Association	Chapter 2
http://www.imia.org/wg1	International Medical Informatics Association	Chapter 2
http://www.vcu.edu/provost/restructuring978/ technologycompetency.html	Virginia Commonwealth University's	Chapter 3

URL	Organizations	Chapter
http://www.utexas.edu/world/lecture/	World Lecture Hall	Chapter 3
http://www.ed.gov/	Department of Education	Chapter 3
http://www.ala.org.	American Library Association	Chapter 3
http://www.ala.org/aasl/ip_nine.html	American Library Association—information literacy standards	Chapter 3
http://www.ala.org/acrl/	Association of College & Research Libraries	Chapter 3
http://www.healthfinder.gov	Healthfinder	Chapter 3
http://www.4women.gov	The National Women's Health Information Center	Chapter 3
http://www.hon.ch/	The Health on the Net Foundation Code of Conduct (HONcode)	Chapter 3
http://www.virginiacolleges.org/exam/frame.html	Virginia Foundation for Independent Colleges (VFIC)	Chapter 3
http://www.hrsa.dhhs.gov/bhpr/DN/nirepex.htm.	National Advisory Council on Nursing Education and Practice—executive summary of a report?	Chapter 3
http://www.ana.org/ancc/index.htm.	American Nurses Credentialing Center	Chapter 3
http://www.ed.gov/pubs/NatAtRisk/title.html.	The National Commission on Excellence in Education (1983). A Nation at Risk: The Imperative for Educational Reform A Report to the Nation and the Secretary of Education United States Department of Education.	Chapter 3

URL	Description	Chapter
http://www.ihc.net/about/mission.html.	Internet Healthcare Coalition, (1998). Mission Statement	Chapter 3
http://www.vcu.edu/provost/restructuring978/technologycompetency.html	Technology Competency of Graduates in Virginia Commonwealth University's Restructuring Report for 1997–98.	Chapter 3
http://www.accrediting-comm-nlnac.org	The National League for Nursing Accrediting Commission	Chapter 3
http://amia-niwg.org	AMIA, Nursing Informatics Workgroup	Chapter 4
http://stats.bls.gov	Department of Labor—Employment Projections.	Chapter 4
http://www.himss.org/himss-member-binaries/compsearch	Healthcare Information and Management Systems Society	Chapter 5
http://www.mllc.org/pedagogy.htm	Middle Level Leadership Center—Pedagogy	Chapter 7
http://www.mllc.org/project.htm	Middle Level Leadership Center—Project Assist	Chapter 7
http://www.duke.edu/~goodw010	Duke University—Linda Goodwin PhD, RN,C	Chapter 7
http://www.microsoft.com	Microsoft	Chapter 7
http://www.real.com	Real Audio	Chapter 7
http://www.lotus.com	Lotus	Chapter 7
http://www.mirabilis.com	ICQ	Chapter 7
http://www.palm.com	Palm Inc.	Chapter 7
http://www.webfayre.com	PenDragon Software Inc.	Chapter 7

URL	Organizations	Chapter
http://www.palm.com	Palm Inc.	Chapter 7
http://www.microsoft.com	Microsoft	Chapter 7
http://home.ubalt.edu/bbrownstein/papers/webteaching.html	Barry Brownstein	Chapter 7
http://www.nlm.nih.gov/pubs/factsheets/trainedu.html	United States National Library of Medicine	Chapter 8
http://www.hl7.org	Health Level 7	Chapter 9
http://aspe.os.hhs.gov/admnsimp	Department of Health and Human Services	Chapter 9
http://www.nursingworld.org/ojin/tpc7/tpc7_2.htm	Nursing World—McCormick, K. & Jones, C.	Chapter 10
http://www.stti.iupui.edu/library	Sigma Theta Tau International—Library	Chapter 11
http://telehealth.hrsa.gov	US Department of Health & Human Services—Information Technology Branch	Chapter 12
http://www.hcfa.gov/medicaid/telelist.htm	Health Care Financing Administration	Chapter 12
http://telehealth.hrsa.gov	Health Resources and Services Administration	Chapter 12
http://www.nlm.nih.gov	National Institutes of Health	Chapter 12
http://www.nasa.gov	National Aeronautics and Space Administration Health and Human Services	Chapter 12

URL	Organizations	Chapter
http://www.healthcare-informatics.com/issues/1999/02_99/nine.htm	Healthcare Informatics Online	Chapter 14
http://ferguson-report.sparklist.com	Ferguson Report	Chapter 14
http://www.med.uni-heidelberg.de/mi.	Institut für Medizinische Biometrie und Informatik—Nightingale Project	Chapter 14
http://www.sgim.org/meetings/am20/ws/infocurric.html.	International Medical Informatics Association	Chapter 14
http://www-iwse.eng.ohio-state.edu/~PJSmith/ITS98.htm	Proceedings of the Forth International Conference on Intelligent Tutoring Systems.	Chapter 14
http://www.sgim.org/meetings/am20/ws/infocurric.html	International Medical Informatics Association	Chapter 14

Index

Page numbers followed by *t* indicate table. Page numbers followed by *f* indicate figure.